THE MARLOWE DIABET

Good control is in your hands.

Since 1999, Marlowe & Company has established itself as the nation's leading independent publisher of books on diabetes. Now, the Marlowe Diabetes Library, launched in 2007, comprises an ever-expanding list of books on how to thrive while living with diabetes or prediabetes. Authors include world-renowned authorities on diabetes and the glycemic index, medical doctors and research scientists, certified diabetes educators, registered dietitians and other professional clinicians, as well as individuals living and thriving with prediabetes, type 1 diabetes, or type 2 diabetes. See page 293 for the complete list of Marlowe Diabetes Library titles.

50 SECRETS

OF THE

ONGEST LIVING PEOPLE

WITH DIABETES

Praise for *50 Secrets of the Longest Living People with Diabetes*

"Inspirational—and practical. A must read that can make a difference in your life."
—Richard N. Podell, M.D., clinical professor, UMDNJ–Robert Wood Johnson Medical School

"*50 Secrets of the Longest Living People with Diabetes* has our hearty recommendation for the inspiration it brings to everyone who desires a long and healthy life."
—John Walsh, P.A., C.D.E., and Ruth Roberts, M.A., authors of *Pumping Insulin* (4th edition), other diabetes books, and www.diabetesnet.com

"The advice that Sheri Colberg and Steven Edelman offer is excellent and will help everyone living with diabetes to live a better, healthier, and longer life . . . Much of their guidance would be well heeded by everyone, not just people with diabetes."
—Jeff Hitchcock, Children with Diabetes

"Information about the inspiring individuals with diabetes was woven in with the fifty great secrets in a very entertaining and educational way. I endorse *50 Secrets of the Longest Living People with Diabetes* to teach, train, and coach those of us with diabetes."
—Paula Harper, R.N., C.D.E., founder and president, Diabetes Exercise & Sports Association

"Most books tell you what the authors think you *should* be doing about your diabetes. *50 Secrets of the World's Longest Living People with Diabetes* tells you what long-lived people with diabetes actually *are* doing about their diabetes . . . Their stories are inspiring as well as instructive."
—Gretchen Becker, author,
The First Year®—Type 2 Diabetes and *Prediabetes*

"While at the University of Michigan we developed the notion of 'patient empowerment' and 'taking control,' which Sheri Colberg and Steven Edeman have captured in a most elegant manner with case histories of people who have thrived for many years despite having diabetes. There is no greater eloquence than that expressed by patients themselves."
—Aaron Vinik, M.D., Ph.D., director,
Strelitz Diabetes Research Center

"Camaraderie is truly what soothes the diabetic breast. As I'm reading read through this book, my neck is getting tired from the constant nodding and saying 'Yes! Yes! This is what it's all about!' Who knows more about living successfully with diabetes than the people who have done it for so many years. After I've soaked up every word, I might be willing to share it with my patients."
—Gary Scheiner, C.D.E., author, *Think Like a Pancreas* and
The Ultimate Guide to Accurate Carb Counting

"*50 Secrets of the Longest Living People with Diabetes* is full of inspiring examples. Sheri Colberg's early belief that she would suffer 'inevitable' consequences of her diabetes struck a particularly strong chord with me . . . Indeed, diabetes is treatable and is more and more treatable all the time, while many other chronic diseases are not. This is another of the excellent and positive points that these two authors make throughout this important book."

—David Mendosa, coauthor, *The New Glucose Revolution What Makes My Blood Glucose Go Up . . . and Down?*, and author, *Losing Weight with Your Diabetes Medication*

"Encouraging, informative, and easy to read . . . this is my kind of diabetes book! If nothing else, you'll be delighted to discover how many of the secrets you've already mastered."

—Amy Tenderich, journalist/blogger, www.diabetesmine.com, and coauthor, *Know Your Numbers, Outlive Your Diabetes*

"*50 Secrets of the Longest Living People with Diabetes* is the Can-Do-est diabetes book you'll ever read. Whatever your age, whatever your current physical and mental health, these vivid experiences of others who've successfully climbed the Diabetes Mountain will inspire you to get on top of the world yourself."

—June Biermann and Barbara Toohey, authors, *The Diabetic's Total Health and Happiness Book*

ABOUT THE AUTHORS

SHERI R. COLBERG, PHD, is an exercise physiologist and associate professor of exercise science at Old Dominion University in Norfolk, Virginia. Having earned a doctorate from the University of California, Berkeley, she specializes in research in diabetes and exercise. She continues to conduct extensive clinical research on diabetes and exercise, with funding from the American Diabetes Association and others. She has also authored myriad articles on exercise and diabetes, as well as three books: *The Diabetic Athlete, Diabetes-Free Kids,* and *The 7 Step Diabetes Fitness Plan.*

Dr. Colberg has almost 40 years of personal experience with type 1 diabetes. Diagnosed with diabetes at the age of 4 in 1968 in what she refers to as the "dark ages" of diabetes care (pre-home blood glucose monitoring), she has spent her life in pursuit of knowledge to allow her to live a healthy life with her disease. She resides in Virginia Beach with her husband and their three boys. An avid recreational exerciser, she enjoys swimming, biking, walking, tennis, weight training, hiking, and yard work, as well as playing with her three sons.

STEVEN V. EDELMAN, MD, an endocrinologist specializing in diabetes care, is a professor at the University of California, San Diego (UCSD) School of Medicine. He directs several programs there and at the VA Medical Center in San Diego. He earned his medical degree at the University of California, Davis School of Medicine, where he was valedictorian of his class, and he completed his internship and residency at UCLA, as well as some additional training during a fellowship at the Joslin Clinic in Boston, among other places.

Diagnosed with diabetes himself at the age of 15, Dr. Edelman has become a local and national leader in diabetes treatment, research, and education. He is founder and director of Taking Control of Your Diabetes (TCOYD), a national not-for-profit organization, as well as the primary author of two books, *Taking Control of Your Diabetes* (3rd edition) and *Diagnosis and Management of Type 2 Diabetes* (6th edition), and the coauthor of at least three more diabetes-related books. When not on the road lecturing and putting on more than ten TCOYD conferences annually, he resides in San Diego with his wife, Ingrid Kruse, a podiatrist who specializes in treatment of diabetic foot problems, and their two teenage daughters.

50 SECRETS

OF THE

ONGEST LIVING PEOPLE

WITH DIABETES

SHERI R. COLBERG, PhD
and
STEVEN V. EDELMAN, MD

MARLOWE DIABETES LIBRARY

MARLOWE & COMPANY

NEW YORK

Copyright © 2007 by Sheri R. Colberg and Steven V. Edelman

Published by
Marlowe and Company
An imprint of Avalon Publishing Group, Incorporated
11 Cambridge Center
Cambridge, MA 02142

AVALON
publishing group incorporated

The information in this book is intended to help readers make informed decisions about their health and the health of their loved ones. It is not intended to be a substitute for treatment by or the advice and care of a professional health-care provider. While the authors and publisher have endeavored to ensure that the information presented is accurate and up-to-date, they shall not be held responsible for loss or damage of any nature suffered as a result of reliance on any of this book's contents or any errors or omissions herein.

Library of Congress Cataloging-in-Publication Data

Colberg, Sheri, 1963-
  50 secrets of the longest living people with diabetes / Sheri R. Colberg
and Steven V. Edelman.
       p. cm.
  Includes bibliographical references.
  ISBN 978-1-60094-018-7 (pbk.)
  1. Diabetes—Popular works. 2. Diabetics—Anecdotes. I. Edelman, Steven
V. II. Title.
RC660.4.C645 2007
616.4'62—dc22

                                    2007014430

9 8 7 6 5 4 3 2

Designed by Maria E. Torres
Printed in the United States of America

For all of the people with diabetes who need a helping hand,
but most of all for Ray Ochs,
my loving husband and supportive partner
in my own diabetes care
—SC

To my loving wife, Ingrid, and my two great kids,
Talia and Carina,
for their never-ending support of my efforts
to help people with diabetes
—SE

CONTENTS

CONCLUSION

INTRODUCTION

FACING THE GHOSTS OF DIABETES PAST, PRESENT, AND FUTURE

Thank goodness that some things are in the past. For instance, one of us (Dr. Sheri Colberg) clearly remembers believing as a preteen that she was doomed to suffer a premature death from diabetic complications before finishing her high school years, at which point she would have already had type 1 diabetes for well over a decade (since the young age of 4). Now, over three decades later and a quarter century past her high school years, she is living well with diabetes, has given birth to three perfectly healthy sons, and has suffered only minor, treatable diabetes complications to date, despite living almost all of her life with the disease.

We consider ourselves the diabetic version of the ghosts of Christmas past, present, and future in Charles Dickens's classic tale, *A Christmas Carol.* As was done for Ebenezer Scrooge, we and many other long-time diabetes survivors are going to help you understand your past, present, and possible future with diabetes—*before* it's too late to change your personal story and choose a different, healthier ending.

PERSONAL GHOSTS OF DIABETES PAST

Luckily for Dr. Sheri, her early beliefs were no more than a Dickens-spawned ghost of diabetes past. Her false assumption of a predestined early demise had arisen from reading on her own about all of the "inevitable" consequences of diabetes, which were admittedly a more common reality before the availability of modern-day management tools, better medications, and a greater understanding of the actual causes of diabetes-related health problems. By finding her way to optimal diabetes control using whatever management tools were available to her at any given point in time, she prevented this possible bad ending from becoming her diabetes present or even a likely future.

"For me, the worst part of getting diabetes when I was 4 was being forced to give up eating Froot Loops!" Dr. Sheri recalls. "Back in 1968 when I was diagnosed with type 1 diabetes (just a month after I had the mumps), the standard diabetes diet required cutting out all sugar. I loved that cereal, and to this day—almost 40 years later—I still remember the cabinet in the kitchen where we used to store the box even though we moved the next year. Getting shots didn't bother me nearly as much as losing my favorite cereal.

"Now, with modern-day insulin analogs and a blood glucose meter, I could eat Froot Loops if I really wanted to and still manage my blood sugars, but to tell you the truth, I tried them once a few years ago and thought they tasted horrible! I don't let my kids eat them either, even though they don't have diabetes, because I know that they make anyone's blood sugar spike rapidly, and no one needs that."

Dr. Steve Edelman's past is a little different from Dr. Sheri's. He didn't develop diabetes until he was already 15 years old. "In junior high school, I would run to the restroom to urinate between classes, relieve my distended bladder, and then slurp up as much water as possible at the drinking fountain," he recalls. "I could not quench my thirst, and all of the kids in line behind me yelled at me because I took so long. Then, halfway through my next class, I would have to urinate again and almost desperately seek out the nearest drinking fountain." He had the classic symptoms of type 1 diabetes. When he finally realized something was really wrong with him, he asked his mother to take him to the doctor, where he was immediately diagnosed.

The ghosts of diabetes past have been more real for Dr. Steve because of his lack of good control in his early years of diabetes. "Every three months I would see my doctor, who would look at my urine and blood glucose results and say the same thing every time. 'Steve, you are doing fine. I will see you next time.' He said the same thing even after I'd had five doughnuts (two glazed, two chocolate cake, and one maple bar) one time before going in for my appointment when I knew my blood sugar was sky-high. In addition, I never went to a camp for diabetic kids or spent any time in support groups or classes for young people with diabetes. I was never educated on how to take an active role in my own diabetes care, and as a result, my control started to slip." Since that time, though, he has sought out the best diabetes care and the knowledge he needs to both control the problems he has (some eye, kidney, and nerve problems) and prevent others from happening, and he regularly shares everything he knows with others.

In retrospect, even Dr. Sheri would agree that giving up eating her favorite sugary cereal, no matter how much it traumatized her at a young age, was well worth the better health she is likely experiencing now by going without eating it. By making other alterations in your diet and lifestyle that are just as simple to implement, you also have the power to change the course of your life and your experience with diabetes. You *can* control your blood glucose levels to prevent diabetes-related health complications from happening to you (or better control any you already have), and in the rest of this book, you'll learn exactly how other long-time diabetes survivors have successfully done it and how you can, too.

IS THE GHOST OF DIABETES PAST IN THE PAST FOR EVERYONE?

Unfortunately, the diabetes past is still all too frequently a part of the present for many people. Poorly controlled diabetes can have a tremendously negative impact on your health. Almost everyone agrees that experiencing good health is truly the most important aspect of living well—with or without diabetes. In fact, without good health, a longer life is not really worth living. If you're unsure, just ask someone with shooting neuropathy pains (due to nerve damage in the feet from diabetes) what he or she would wish for: a longer life or a pain-free one. While it's perfectly understandable to wish for both a long *and* a healthy life (most of us desire both), if forced to make a choice between living long and living well, almost all of us would choose having good health for the rest of our lives, with living longer as our secondary goal.

When diabetes enters the picture, though, you could lose out on both counts. Diabetes has the potential to rob you, on average, of more than twelve years of your life. What's more, it can also dramatically reduce your quality of life for more than twenty of those years by negatively impacting your health while you are still alive. Your quality of life can be reduced by many physical ailments, but diabetes often causes disability through partial limb amputations, chronic pain, loss of mobility, blindness, chronic dialysis, and/or heart disease. In fact, experts recently estimated that for the 38.5 percent of average females born in the year 2000 or later predicted to develop diabetes, the disease will shorten their lives by over 14 years (if diagnosed by the age of 40) and make their lives a lot less worth living during the last 22. As diabetes survivors ourselves, we can't think of anything *less* desirable than living a shorter, disease-limited life.

Just by having diabetes, you already have twice the risk of dying young as someone who is diabetes-free. If you're a younger type 2 diabetic person (between 25 and 44 years old), your risk is almost four times as high. Diabetes is the sixth leading cause of death, but it should actually have a higher ranking. For instance, if you die from a heart attack or stroke, your death certificate may not even mention diabetes as a cause or contributing factor, even though we now know that poor blood sugar control accelerates the blockage of arteries around your body. The World Health Organization recently estimated that diabetes kills more people worldwide than previously thought, causing well more than 3.2 million deaths per year, or at least six deaths from diabetes every minute of each and every day.

THE RAPIDLY GROWING DIABETES PRESENT

We're not dwelling on the darker side of diabetes to upset you. Rather, our goal is to give you hope for a brighter future by increasing your awareness of what's possible and how to prevent problems. Without better education and a concerted effort, all the diabetes management tools in the world aren't going to make a difference or keep the diabetes past out of our collective present and future lives. The world is currently experiencing the fastest rise in cases of diabetes ever, resulting in an epidemic all around the globe. In fact, American children born in the new millennium have a one in three chance of developing diabetes in their lifetime, and for many minorities like Hispanics and African-Americans, the risk is closer to one in two. Likely more than 21 million people in the United States already have diabetes (7 percent of the entire population), although a third of them still have no idea that they do, and every twenty-one seconds someone is diagnosed with it. A recent conservative prediction of the number of diabetic Americans in the year 2030 is that there will be over 30 million, but with the way things are currently going, it's likely to be much higher.

More than 90 percent of people are developing type 2 diabetes, which is largely due to an interaction of genetics and lifestyle habits that result in insulin resistance. In their bodies, the glucose-lowering hormone insulin is unable to effectively manage blood sugars, and they usually end up losing too many pancreatic beta cells to make enough insulin, so they will often have to take insulin injections to make up the difference. Another 5 to 10 percent have type 1 diabetes, which results from an abnormal immune system response (and possibly altered sensory nerves) that wipes out their bodies' own beta cells, leaving them dependent on external insulin for the rest of their lives. Like type 2s, though, people with type 1 diabetes can also develop an insulin-resistant state as a result of lifestyle choices, which only makes their diabetes harder to control. So, when it comes right down to it, no matter what type of diabetes you have, the secrets to controlling it, living well, and preventing diabetes-related health complications are remarkably similar, as you are soon going to find out.

A SWIFTLY CHANGING GHOST OF DIABETES FUTURE?

Despite current remaining obstacles to diabetes prevention and control, the future of diabetes is still looking brighter and brighter all the time. The message we want to convey to you is that you can take control of your diabetes, even if you already have complications. It is never too late to feel in control, both mentally and physically. Reaching this future starts with learning from the lessons offered by survivors of past years with diabetes. Many long-time diabetic survivors have been officially identified and awarded by the Joslin Diabetes Center, Lilly Pharmaceuticals, and others. The Joslin facility was started as a private practice in 1898 by Elliott P. Joslin, MD, who believed that the key to managing diabetes is patient involvement, education, and empowerment. This philosophy closely parallels the one that Dr. Steve has adopted for his educational, not-for-profit organization, Taking Control of Your Diabetes (TCOYD), which puts on conferences and health fairs around the country as part of his mission (www.tcoyd.org).

Some time ago, researchers began to track long-living people with diabetes to find out their secrets of longevity. For example, in 1970, the Joslin Diabetes Center established the 50-Year Medal, an award given to anyone using insulin to treat diabetes for a half century (to correspond with 50 years of insulin availability starting in 1921), and they are also studying these individuals to find out their longevity secrets. As of 2005, more than 2,200 people worldwide had received this medal. On the seventy-fifth anniversary of the discovery of insulin in 1996, they also awarded the first medal for living 75 years with diabetes, and as of 2005, over sixteen people had been recognized for achieving this remarkable feat. Lilly Pharmaceuticals, the original manufacturer of insulin for diabetic use (but now just one of several companies that make it), also established 25-, 50-, and 75-year awards (for insulin users) as part of its LillyforLife program in 1974, and since the program's inception, this company has presented more than 1,500 of its own 50-Year Insulin Awards. While the majority of the recognized individuals have type 1 diabetes, anyone with type 2 diabetes who has been using insulin for at least a quarter of a century also qualifies for these awards.

What makes these long-living individuals' accomplishments so remarkable is that blood glucose meters have only been widely available since the early 1980s, so these survivors have lived a large part of their diabetic lives without the benefit of knowing their exact blood glucose readings (or being able to fully control them). Furthermore, the average life span for most individuals, with diabetes or without, is only around 74 years for men and 78 years for women in the United States, so living for 75 years with the disease means that they have outlived many people living without it.

Through his contact with thousands of conference attendees yearly throughout the United States, Dr. Steve has also met many other motivated individuals who have lived long and well despite having diabetes. Most of them have type 1 diabetes, formerly known as juvenile diabetes because its onset is most common in children and adolescents. However, many of them are also long-living people with type 2 diabetes. The lessons learned from both are similar and apply to everyone, their key secret being that strict control of your blood sugars can help prevent diabetic complications, regardless of the type of diabetes you have.

"I wish my doctor during my teenage years had given me better advice on the benefits of controlling my blood sugars. I have my diabetes under control now, but all of those early years of being in less than good control have taken a toll on my body," Dr. Steve remarks. "If I had only known then what I know now, I probably wouldn't be having any problems with my health after almost 38 years with diabetes." He currently takes medications to protect his kidney function, and so far he's doing well despite having been diagnosed with kidney disease almost 20 years ago. "I know that my better blood sugars are also a key factor in keeping my body in good shape now and for the next 40 years . . . or more."

The really good news is that although having any type of diabetes requires you to follow a rigorous set of daily tasks and choices to control it effectively, doing so has become vastly easier in the last quarter century due to the wide availability of new management tools and cutting-edge diabetic medications and technologies, including rapid-acting insulin analogs, new medications for the treatment of both type 1 and type 2 diabetes, a plethora of blood glucose monitors, and even continuous glucose-monitoring devices as of 2006. As a result, millions of people now have access to everything they need to manage their diabetes successfully and to live long and complication-free lives. The best suggestion is to follow the advice of Rabbi Hirsch Meisels of Spring Valley, New York, who says, "Focus on the present and the future, and don't dwell on the past." It's good to realize how far we've come, but it's more important to take charge of your diabetes now, with the hope of even better treatments and tools or a cure in the not-too-distant future.

A SHORT TALE ABOUT TWO LONG DIABETIC LIVES

Few people so far have managed as well or as long as the Cleveland brothers of Syracuse, New York, who have over 157 years of living with diabetes between them. Robert "Bob" Cleveland, reaching his 87th birthday in March of 2007, has lived longer with diabetes than almost anyone else so far—82 years—since the age of 5, just a few years after the discovery of insulin in 1921. Even more remarkable, though, is the fact that he is not the sole member of his family who has survived a remarkably long time with diabetes. His older brother, Gerald, who turned 91 years old in January, has also had type 1 diabetes since childhood—only slightly less long at 75 years, since the age of 16. Experts say that they know of no other person who has lived to be as old as Gerald after having had type 1 diabetes most of his life.

While inheriting a good set of family genes undoubtedly has something to do with the extended longevity of these brothers, there is far more to it than just that. Scientists tracking the brothers and other long-living diabetes survivors say that while these remarkable individuals almost certainly have some genetic advantages, what has helped them just as much are their underlying behaviors in controlling their disease: vigilance, hard work, self-sacrifice, and determination. Both brothers have meticulously kept track of their blood glucose readings, insulin doses, diet, and exercise on a daily basis for most of their diabetic years. In their early lives with diabetes, times were quite different, and all they could really do at that time was to be vigilant and hope for the best. The Clevelands have actually lived most of their lives in what we often refer to as the "dark ages" of diabetes care (including decades of even "darker" years than both of us have lived through). Before the early 1980s, almost no one had access to the modern tools of diabetes care, like home blood glucose monitors and synthetic human insulins, to help optimize control of blood sugars. The expected outcomes of diabetes back then included amputations, blindness, kidney failure, and heart disease, not to mention a severely shortened life span.

The Cleveland brothers were lucky to develop diabetes just late enough to have insulin commercially available and be able to survive those early years and many, many more. At the time that they were born (1916 and 1920), type 1 diabetes was still a death sentence within weeks or months in most cases (even on a "starvation" diet with limited carbohydrate and food intake) because insulin was not discovered until 1921, and it was not widely available commercially until 1922 to 1923, mostly in the larger suburban areas. Likewise, although type 2 diabetes could often be controlled with diet and exercise, it also usually led to years of debilitating illness and a shortened life expectancy. Just a few years after the brothers' arrival into the world, however, scientists at the University of Toronto isolated insulin in a form that was effective and safe enough for human use (although far from optimal), and then Eli Lilly & Company began to mass-produce it for the first time by 1922. Although insulin's discovery kept the 5-year-old Gerald from dying soon after his diagnosis in 1925, it didn't change the fact that he had a difficult road with diabetes ahead of him. Admittedly, controlling diabetes was hard and painful work back in the early decades of insulin therapy, and the good control of today was simply not possible to achieve like it is nowadays.

In the early years, insulin was made from pancreases of pigs and cows and was so impure that the doses needed were many times larger than typical ones today. What's more, the insulin's strength was often inconsistent. Even when the product became purer and more predictable, some people suffered serious adverse reactions to it. The insulins were also only short-acting ones that had to be given frequently to cover both meals and basal insulin needs. Moreover, people using these insulins did not have any way to measure their actual blood glucose levels, and as a result, they often suffered from a roller-coaster ride of damaging blood sugar highs and dangerous lows. Until the development in 1936 of a longer-acting insulin (PZI) that stabilized insulin levels throughout the day and night, doctors advised patients to interrupt their sleep to inject themselves rather than let their sugar levels climb through the night from lack of insulin. Human synthetic insulins were not available until Lilly got FDA approval for the first one (Humulin) in 1982.

Even up until about twenty-five years ago (almost six decades into Bob Cleveland's time with diabetes), the only tool people had to use at home to get some feedback on their blood sugar levels was an antiquated method of testing urine for glucose, which was notoriously inaccurate. For decades, the Clevelands and millions of other people with diabetes (including both Dr. Sheri and Dr. Steve) caught their urine in cups and then added a chemical reactant to a certain amount of urine diluted with water that turned it various colors depending on the amount of sugar in it, running the gamut from dark blue (indicating sugar-free urine) to bright orange for the highest concentration of sugar that could be measured.

Of course, this method was still a more accurate technique for determining blood sugar levels than was available in even earlier times. In the second century AD, during Greek times, the name "diabetes," meaning "siphon," was adopted to describe patients with great thirst and excessive urination, and in the seventeenth century, the term "mellitus" (meaning "like honey") was added to describe the sweet smell of their sugar-filled urine. Reportedly, physicians back in those days tasted urine for sugar content to diagnose the disease, but we're sure that it wasn't an accurate way to measure the actual quantity present!

Being aggressive about controlling diabetes back in the Cleveland brothers' early years meant running a serious risk of taking too much insulin, which could easily have resulted in a hypoglycemic coma and early death. The alternative, though, was to let their blood glucose levels stay higher than normal, which over many years could lead to damage and the potential for many diabetic complications. We're happy to report, however, that against these immense odds, both of the Cleveland brothers have had successful careers, long marriages, children, grandchildren, and great-grandchildren—with truly a minimum of diabetes-related health problems. In fact, 91-year-old Gerald believes that he has lived as long as he has so he can help inspire others with the disease. "My main reason to stay alive is to prove to young people there's a way to live with diabetes, to live well," he says.

Now, as diabetes poses a rapidly rising threat to the health of so many Americans and others worldwide, the remarkable lives of these brothers offer the ultimate diabetic success story, giving all of us hope that living a long and healthy life with diabetes is a real possibility for everyone. Thankfully, long gone are the days when diabetic complications and a shortened life span were a foregone conclusion, a sentence that was handed down along with the diagnosis. The Clevelands have lived long and generally healthy lives in part through extraordinary discipline in diet, exercise, and monitoring of their diabetes, along with a very positive outlook on life.

The discipline involved in living well for so long has not always been easy. As Bob admits, "I never had any sweets as a child—never." Even to this day, his older brother Gerald keeps meticulous logs of his insulin doses and blood sugar readings, tests his sugars seven or more times a day, avoids desserts and rapidly absorbed starches, exercises, and stays thin. Gerald is still a compulsive reader of food ingredient labels, so he knows exactly what is going into his body and how much insulin it's going to take. Both brothers still recognize the importance of their diet and daily exercise in living well. At 87, Bob is still an avid cyclist, often biking twenty or more miles outdoors, while Gerald regularly attends exercise classes and does daily exercises with five-pound weights. Largely due to their extraordinary diligence, the brothers' lives have been even longer than the average life span for most people and remarkably free of any serious diabetic complications.

Both of the Clevelands have developed some of the circulatory and nerve problems in the feet that are so common to people with diabetes, but just in recent years (after a very long time with diabetes and no access to blood glucose meters during most of their lives). Gerald has also undergone several operations for "trigger finger," a condition most prevalent in people with diabetes that causes curved fingers that can't be unbent without surgery. Nevertheless, these complications are relatively minor, and both continue to make a point of meeting with younger people with diabetes, giving them hope and encouragement. "It hasn't been easy," Gerald says, "but I've had a terrific life."

WHAT THE FUTURE HOLDS FOR YOU

Likely, no one reading this book will have lived as long with diabetes as Bob and Gerald Cleveland (with the exception of Gladys Dull—more on her to come in the first profile), but it's a goal that we can all aspire to reach. Initially, the idea for this book came about when the story of the Cleveland brothers' long lives with diabetes was picked up by the media early in 2006 (specifically the *New York Times*), which brought a greater public awareness to the fact that people really can live a long time and in good health despite having diabetes. At some point in our lives since our diagnoses, we have all invariably turned to others with more diabetes experience like the Clevelands for advice and support. Maybe you have done the same not just for yourself, but on behalf of your diabetic child, significant other, or aging parent. Regardless of the circumstances under which diabetes has entered into your life, you can learn from other people living with diabetes, even if they have had it for a shorter time. The people interviewed for this book really have a handle on what works and what doesn't. What's more, they're beyond willing to share what they know to help you also live a long and healthy life with diabetes.

With the intent of taking advantage of this wealth of experience, we conducted well over fifty interviews with people living with both type 1 and type 2 diabetes. They range in age from 34 to 93 years "young" and have experienced from 19 to more than 83 years of living with and managing the disease using any and all tools available at the time. Close to 40 percent have lived with diabetes for 50 or more years, and two-thirds have amassed at least four decades' worth of diabetes experience. Most are insulin users (even the long-living type 2s), but even if you are not currently using insulin, 99 percent of the information in this book still directly applies to you and your diabetes control. In addition to sifting out the gems from these many interviews, we pulled supporting information from the latest, relevant research studies and educational articles, along with tapping into the knowledge of diabetes professionals like ourselves and others.

The result is a list of fifty of the most important and commonly given "secrets," advice and suggestions that you can easily incorporate into your lifestyle to optimize your blood sugars and prevent diabetes complications. Admittedly, there are still others, but we had to exclude some to condense the book down to a more manageable size. For example, we were forced to cut out a few that came up less often and may not be relevant to everyone, such as, "Don't vary your diet." Eating a variety of foods has become more feasible nowadays with the advent of blood glucose meters, newer insulins, and other medications that more effectively control blood sugars before and after meals when you choose to include differing types and amounts of food. In other words, these secrets are as up-to-date and universally relevant to everyone with diabetes (even diabetes during pregnancy, or gestational) as possible.

In the coming chapters, you will additionally read many stories about these diabetes survivors, along with their personal secrets of longevity and advice that can help you to live a longer, healthier, more fulfilling life with diabetes, too. Even if you adopt only some of the key suggestions given in this book, your future with diabetes has the potential to be even brighter than it has been for many of the interviewees, especially given all the amazing advances in diabetes care that are now available to you. In addition, nine in-depth profiles of some amazing long-living individuals with diabetes are sure to inspire you, starting with the following story of Gladys Dull, who has remarkably lived long and well with diabetes since 1924. Read on to take your future into your own hands once and for all.

GLADYS C. LESTER DULL, AGE 90, LIVING WITH TYPE 1 DIABETES FOR 83 YEARS

Although the Cleveland brothers' joint longevity is impressive, a woman equally deserving of admiration is Gladys Dull, a Walla Walla, Washington resident since 1938 who has been on insulin injections just slightly longer than Bob Cleveland has—since November of 1924, a couple of months before she turned 7 years old. To our knowledge, she is the longest-living person with diabetes to date.

Born in North Dakota, she lost her birth parents during a flu epidemic in 1920 when she was only 3 years old. Fortunately, she and one of her sisters were soon adopted and raised by some neighbors who were part of the farming community there. She remembers feeling sick before her diagnosis and needing to urinate all the time. After traveling the nine miles from where they lived in the country to the nearest doctor, she was diagnosed with diabetes, but the small-town doctor didn't know how to treat it. He suggested that her adoptive parents take her to the Mayo Clinic in Rochester, Minnesota, which they consented to do. Gladys remembers the long train trip from her home to the clinic, where she was immediately admitted to the hospital for treatment with the newly available, Lilly-made insulin.

"I remember the first shot I got and being scared of it," Gladys recalls more than eight decades later. "The needles back then were a lot more painful than they are now—and a lot more expensive." Her mother had to go to classes at the Mayo Clinic to learn what to do for her, including weighing wax figures of food that were a certain number of grams. "My mother weighed everything out for me after that," she says. "She'd let me have one gram more than what I was supposed to have." Since she wasn't allowed to eat candy anymore, her grandfather used to buy her a newspaper to read (for the comics) instead, which almost made up for the one piece of candy a week she used to get on a trip into town.

Gladys has enjoyed the support of family and friends for all of her life with diabetes, including her husband, George Dull, with whom she enjoyed a 59-year marriage that ended in 2002 with his passing. Married in 1943 during WWII, she and her husband (who was born in 1915) were separated for two and a half years while he was stationed overseas with his Army unit. Later, after his return, they moved to Walla Walla, where she has lived ever since and worked part-time in a portrait studio for 30 years. At the age of 30, she gave birth to her only child, Norm Dull, who lives in a nearby town in Washington State. Amazingly, she has outlived all four of her brothers and sisters, two of whom were older, the other two younger, and all diabetes-free. Her last sister recently died from Alzheimer's disease (of which Gladys has absolutely no signs, even though the risk is possibly higher in people with diabetes). "After seeing what my sister went through, I would much rather be diabetic than have Alzheimer's," Gladys says.

This spunky 90-year-old with diabetes attributes most of her success to being active most of her life and to sticking to her diet. "When I was younger, I did everything—horseback riding, cycling, snowmobiling, motorcycle riding—I always stayed active." In addition, because of her early training, to this day Gladys can still tell approximately how much a serving of any food weighs, and she still watches her portions strictly. "I give my mother credit for that," she says. "She was strict with me, and I thank her for it now." Her son also credits Gladys with raising him on her diet, saying, "I still eat lots of veggies, thanks to Mom." Her diet doesn't vary much, and neither do her insulin requirements.

In all likelihood, another of her secrets is the fact that she has religiously taken her insulin shots since they first saved her life back in 1924. "I have never missed a shot in all these years," she affirms. "To date, I've had over 60,000 of them." Taking injections is just a small price to pay for her longevity, though. May we all strive to live so long and do so well with diabetes!

The 50 Secrets

PART ONE

Emotional Secrets

1

Live First and Be Diabetic Second

A key secret to being successful with diabetes is to first and foremost live a normal life. "Being diabetic is as much a psychological and spiritual experience as it is a physical condition," says Don Gifford of Columbia, Maryland, who has lived with diabetes for 52 years already (since the age of 2). Judy Tripathi of Bryn Mawr, Pennsylvania, who works as a diabetes educator at Integrated Diabetes Services in Wynnewood, agrees with Don (as do most other long-living survivors) that diabetes is as much or more about your philosophy as it is about medicine. "Live first, and be a diabetic second," she advises. Judy has been living with diabetes for 43 years since the age of 12 and says that one of her biggest secrets has been to find a healthy balance between giving enough attention to her diabetes control without becoming obsessive about it. Certainly, "living first" doesn't mean that diabetes should be ignored; it simply means that having diabetes should not be the overwhelming focus of your life.

To be politically and psychologically correct, you really shouldn't ever be called a "diabetic" (used as a noun), but rather a "person with diabetes" to change the focus away from identifying your whole persona with having a chronic disease. Luckily for Patty Chambers Schaeffer, a resident of Virginia Beach, Virginia, who has lived with diabetes for 70 of her 73 years, her parents didn't make a big deal about her diabetes. "I had blue eyes, brown hair, and diabetes," she recounts. "It was just a part of my life." Vena Petrotta, a 71-year-old, almost 60 year veteran of diabetes who lives in Hampton, Virginia, agrees. "You have to live a normal life." Also living with diabetes for 60 years since the age of 12, Peter Gariti of Williamsburg, Virginia, echoes a similar thought. "Diabetes is constantly with you. You have to be aware of it, but don't dwell on it and get depressed," he advises. "You can live a long time and a good life with diabetes." A resident of San Diego, California, Grant McArthur also says one of his secrets of living well with diabetes for 42 of his 63 years is that he has "lived a pretty good life." Diabetes has certainly been an acknowledged part of it, but not his primary focus.

For Marialice Kern, who lives in Concord, California (in the San Francisco Bay area), learning not to take diabetes so seriously that it changed her life was important. "You have to go about what you normally do," she advises after living with diabetes for 32 of her 50 years. A Portland, Oregon, resident, Chuck Eichten has felt that one of his barriers has just been balancing a "normal life" with the real constraints of having diabetes for 31 years, since the age of 14. He has always strived to live first, be diabetic second, but he found in college it was difficult. "I remember everyone else in college having random eating habits—like the occasional pizza at 2:00 AM—and sleeping until noon, but I just couldn't do it. At the time, he was still only on one shot of insulin a day, and that regimen wasn't very flexible. (If he could attend college over again with today's blood glucose meters, insulin pumps, and newer insulins, he may well be able to fully live first and worry about having diabetes more as an afterthought.)

Paul McGuigan, a 50-year-old resident of South Euclid, Ohio, living with diabetes for the second half of his life, says that you can't let diabetes get to you. "It's a chronic illness," he says, "so you have to treat it chronically. Treat it, and then go on with your life." He prefers positive statements like "let's just do it" and "move forward" to negative ones like "poor me."

2

Keep a Positive Attitude

Speaking of positive statements, many long-living people with diabetes are adamant that having a positive attitude is one of the key secrets to living well with diabetes, avoiding depression, and feeling happy overall, and research supports their assertion. In support of their belief, a recent 40-year study following students initially studied at the University of North Carolina at Chapel Hill in the mid-1960s found that pessimists had a 42 percent higher death rate from all causes compared with optimists. Individuals with the sunnier outlooks were less likely to suffer from depression, and the link between this mental condition and a lesser physical well-being is well established.

A more positive outlook can result from many influences, including good support from family and friends, a conscious choice to look for the silver lining in every situation, and for some, a strong faith. "Be grateful for the whole package," say Don Gifford, by way of example, "and realize that you are extraordinarily fortunate for what you have." Many chronic diseases are not treatable, but diabetes is, and the treatments available today are better than ever and advancing at a rapid rate. "My perspective now produces a feeling of everyday good fortune," Don states. "I thank God I'm alive and healthy." Chuck Eichten echoes Don's sentiments, saying, "Unlike with a lot of other chronic diseases, you at least have some control over diabetes. I always felt empowered and never developed a negative attitude about it. It's not like being diagnosed with brain cancer." Even after having had diabetes since 1924, Gladys Dull still would choose it over other diseases. "I lost my last sister to Alzheimer's disease in September 2006. She had gotten so bad that she slept all day and then got up and wandered outside at night. I would much rather be a diabetic. I just hope I'll be able to keep doing what I do now."

When Karen Poenisch of Avon, Indiana, found out she had diabetes at the age of 8 almost 43 years ago, she knew nothing about it, which is not uncommon. She remembers that when the doctors at the hospital in Phoenix (where she lived growing up) initially told her she had the disease, she thought she was going to die. When they explained to her that she wasn't going to die, but would have to take a shot every day for the rest of her life, she said, "Well, it's better than dying." To this day, she believes that keeping a positive attitude is vital to living well with diabetes. "You have to accept having diabetes and find out what you need to know to keep it under control," she states. "I've been open to trying a lot of things in my life that can help. You can't ignore diabetes, or it kills you." As a diabetes educator, she has seen many people who have had it for years and who were not doing well. On the whole, though, the people she saw who tried hard to accept and control their diabetes did much better.

Encinitas, California, resident Larry Verity had a similar response to developing diabetes at the age of 23, over 30 years ago. "My diagnosis was a total shock," he said. "I was working on my master's degree at the University of Virginia at the time. But I remember thinking that I could have a lot worse things than diabetes." Similarly, a 66-year-old resident of San Diego, California, Will Speer, Sr., has been living with diabetes for the past 39 years, but he doesn't remember ever feeling depressed about it. In fact, like Larry, he feels lucky that he *only* has diabetes, even though when he was diagnosed at the age of 27, the only advice he got from his doctor was to "go have a good time because you only have five years to live." He says, "I go to the VA Hospital, and I see people with much worse problems. I also have two half-brothers with diabetes. One just lay around and complained about diabetes until he died from its complications, and the other one lives on candy bars and Pepsi. He's still alive and in his 70s, but he has had heart attacks and other problems. I just try to do the best I can."

Anna Maria Gould, who was born and raised (and still lives) in San Antonio, Texas, has maintained a positive attitude for the past 42 years since being diagnosed with diabetes at the age of 9. "I try to stay positive. I'm proactive, too, and I try to prevent problems with my diabetes and get back on track right away. I really think you've got to accept the disease and learn to live with it." S. Fasten from Brooklyn, New York, was diagnosed at the age of 4 and has lived with diabetes for 37 years already. He also agrees that you have to have "a very healthy, happy attitude" to be successful with diabetes over the long haul. Rabbi Meisels, who has been living with diabetes for over 27 years (since the age of 5), agrees: "Stay positive! Talk positive about your diabetes and yourself."

Dan Spinazzola, a resident of Solana Beach, California, who has been living with type 2 diabetes for almost the last 20 of his 68 years, recognizes the importance of being upbeat about diabetes as well. "I try to be positive about everything in my life. I'll also try everything that might help," he says, which means that he's willing to follow his doctor's (who just happens to be Dr. Steve) advice about new medications or regimens he should try to better control his diabetes. "I work hard at it," he admits, but he doesn't let it get him down. Matt Besley, a 24-year veteran of diabetes who lives in Carlsbad, California, says that staying positive for him means having a feeling that something better or a cure is out there—in the near future. He developed diabetes at the age of 10, so he has a lot of living with diabetes left to do.

If anyone has a reason not to feel that positive, it would be Patricia La France-Wolf from Temple City, California, who has been living with diabetes for 63 years since the tender age of 22 months. Instead of being negative, though, she says, "Diabetes doesn't have to ruin your life. If you have a good attitude, everything in your diet, exercise, and medicine goes better." She should know, especially since she has had to deal with being blind from diabetic eye complications for the past 30 years. She obviously practices what she preaches, given that her number one secret for diabetes longevity is to "have a good attitude." Until just recently, she worked for the California State Department of Rehabilitation teaching newly blind people how to live well despite their disability. Even in retirement, she continues to volunteer and teach diabetes education classes for the blind. In 2006, in recognition of her remarkable life, she was the honored recipient of the Lillyfor-Life Achievement Award in the "Adult Achiever" category.

A resident of Goldsboro, North Carolina, Carol Sessions has lived with diabetes since 1960 (a total of 47 years) since she was only 3 years old. For her and many others, spiritual belief has been an important part of keeping a positive outlook and doing well with her diabetes. She also advises, "Don't get too discouraged, and don't give up!" Karen Poenisch agrees with her. "Having a strong faith in God has helped me," she says. "When I was having trouble figuring out how to control my blood sugars before I became pregnant, I asked the Lord to show me how to do it. When I was in the shower, an explanation came forth, and I was able to do it and get pregnant." Anna Maria Gould also feels that her faith has really pulled her through. "My mom was told when I was diagnosed at the age of 9 that I wouldn't make it to 15," she says. "Because of my early experiences, it's now a mission in my life to try to help a lot of people with diabetes. I give thanks to God for being there for me."

Along the same lines, when listing her secrets of living 41 of her 51 years well with diabetes, Jane Dohrmann, a resident of Norfolk, Virginia, listed faith and attitude as her top two. "There has to be faith in order to live with any chronic illness," she says. "I don't think I could have made it this far without it." As for her attitude, she adds, "I have always done my very best to keep my attitude a positive one." In fact, there have been studies showing that your attitude has a lot to do with how you'll heal after surgery or recover from a serious illness. As Gerald Cleveland says after 75 years of living with the disease and over 70 years of active involvement with his church, "I still look forward to the next day more than the last." May we all be so positive the rest of our days!

Depression is a real problem for many people living with diabetes, though, and one that is best prevented or effectively treated. In some cases, researchers believe that depression may lead to the onset of diabetes, rather than the other way around, which may be largely explainable by the effects of cortisol, a natural hormone that decreases the action of insulin in your body. People who are depressed generally have higher cortisol levels in their bloodstreams throughout the day, and their coping skills may be minimal when they're feeling that way, meaning that they'll be less likely to take good care of their bodies. Depression can also make you more likely to seek comfort in foods or behaviors that can contribute to the onset of diabetes or worsen your control.

If you're prone to feeling "blue," you may want to make yourself become more optimistic instead by practicing strategies like anger management and meditation to boost positive emotions. In a study of Tibetan Buddhist monks, many who have spent over 10,000 hours of their lives in meditation, researchers found evidence that a positive state of mind is a skill that can be trained, much as the monks accomplish with hours of focused thought. It appears that the conscious act of thinking about your thoughts in a particular way can rearrange your brain. If nothing else, putting on a sunny face regardless of how you really feel can actually alter your mood for the better by affecting your thought patterns.

🦚 3 🦚

Refuse to Be a Victim

You are the only one with the capacity to change your thoughts and attitudes for the better. Thankfully, you have the power to change how you view any situation or occurrence in your life, including the onset of diabetes. While it would be easy for anyone with diabetes to feel depressed over the fact that it's currently an incurable condition, you're much more likely to have a good life despite having diabetes if you positively set out to use all the tools and information at your disposal to control your blood glucose levels to the best of your ability. At least then you'd be taking positive steps to control the things that you *can* influence and letting go of the things that you *can't*.

As soon as you regard yourself as a victim of diabetes, you're likely to become ineffective at taking control of your diabetes and truly become one, in a self-fulfilling prophecy sort of way. Long-living diabetes survivors have climbed mountains, traveled and flown airplanes solo around the world, done many more amazing feats, and lived long and healthy lives, all because they refused to let diabetes keep them from doing anything or from taking care of themselves.

"Don't let anyone tell you that you can't do something because of diabetes," Don Gifford advises. "Don't view yourself as a victim of diabetes. As soon as you regard yourself as one, you're done." Obviously, he hasn't allowed himself to become a diabetes victim since he has climbed mountains, gone to law school, and raised a family. Peter Gariti has also lived a long and industrious life with diabetes, working many years for General Electric in various locations around the country. "I remember after I got diabetes when I was 12, my dad said to me that having diabetes is good because it will make me learn to take better care of myself, that I would benefit by learning how to be healthy throughout my life." At 72 and still going strong six decades later, Peter agrees that his father's words had a positive impact on how he viewed his diabetes from the start.

Although 65-year-old Rich Humphreys of Kirkwood, Pennsylvania, has had diabetes for more than 51 years, he has also refused to let it slow him down, regardless of the hurdles it occasionally set up in his life. A testament to his determination, he started working to set up a nature trail for kids (along which they could look for gnomes, as well as learn about protecting the environment) when he started losing his eyesight from diabetic retinopathy. He had been an art teacher, but he realized that without his sight, there was no way he would be able to continue in that line of employment. The good news is that although he lost his sight completely in one eye for over a year, he now has it fully restored in both eyes. One of his main secrets is to "see life as an adventure and have fun." Similarly, Al Lewis, a retired oceanography professor who has lived with diabetes for 69 of his 73 years, says that diabetes affected his outlook some, but mostly it was "just there." He never let it keep him from ocean fishing as a teenager, scuba diving as an adult, or any other pursuit he was interested in.

Bob Elder of Southern Shores, North Carolina, says one of his secrets of living 46 of his 69 years with diabetes and without complications is to not dwell on it. "I hate using diabetes as an excuse for anything," he says. "You can't ever forget about it, though. I'm always conscious of the fact that I'm limited in that respect." He just doesn't let it keep him from enjoying life, doing what he wants to do, and staying active.

"I haven't done anything unusual with my life," claims Carolyn Balcom of Sterling, Virginia, who has had diabetes for 43 of her 72 years. "I have never let diabetes keep me from doing anything I wanted to do, though." She has raised five kids (three of her own and two foster children) and now has seven grandchildren. "When I went back to work when my kids were in school, I worked as a night shift nurse for the next 25 years, and I learned how to adjust my insulin to that schedule." Similarly, Natalie Saunders, a resident of Virginia Beach, Virginia, living with diabetes for 36 years since the age of 32, says that she doesn't let diabetes stop her or even slow her down. "I go and I do. I travel—I've been to Israel and Paris—I do whatever," she states.

Jane Dohrmann also talks of the courage it takes to deal with having diabetes or any other illness. "When going through things that are new and unknown, somewhere deep down in your soul you have to search for courage." Related to that concept, she also feels that determination is a key to success. "There are things in every diabetic person's life that require a 'go-get-um' approach," she says. "I think it's one of those factors that is similar to 'stubborn,' but holds a different tone."

The most remarkable story of someone who is anything but a victim, though, is about Marc Blatstein, a 47-year veteran of diabetes (since the age of 10) and a resident of Huntington Valley, Pennsylvania. He credits diabetes with saving his life. On April 29, 1984, when he was just 34 years old, he and his cousin drove to a warehouse to move a woodturning lathe, weighing approximately 2000 pounds, for his cousin's brother. Both Marc and his cousin lifted weights, were in excellent physical shape, and weighed in at 245 pounds, so the task was an easy one for them. Their mission accomplished, Marc headed off to find a restroom, but things did not go as planned. While walking through a dark room in the warehouse that was on his way, Marc tripped and fell backward down through a trapdoor that had accidentally been left open, landing on his back on solid concrete 21 feet below. The result was that he was so badly injured—his back was broken in three places, most of his ribs were broken, he couldn't feel his lower extremities, and he had massive internal injuries—that he was not expected to live.

In the ambulance on the way to the emergency room, Marc recalls, "I heard one of the paramedics say, 'I don't think he's gonna make it.' At that point, I thought to myself, 'That's what you think, buddy.' I still had my life ahead of me, my wife, and my children. Damn it, I wasn't gonna die that day!" After making it through some surgeries, lung trauma (when he almost drowned as his lungs filled up with blood), and a prognosis of only regaining limited movement in his lower extremities (but not the ability to walk), he proved all the doctors wrong. Needless to say, it was a long, hard road back; one that involved two weeks on life support, months and months of traction, body casts, body braces, physical rehab, and Marc's iron will to walk and function normally again, but in the end, he eventually regained his ability to do everything he had been able to before his accident.

Marc clearly remembers one visit he had from an endocrinologist after he did the impossible and starting moving his legs again enough to take a step. The doctor said to Marc's parents, "Your son has survived a major accident and come very far in a short period of time. His rehabilitation has been moved forward tremendously because of his positive attitude and emotional fortitude. The reason Marc has survived this accident is because he has diabetes." By way of explanation, the doctor stated that diabetes had made Marc a stronger person, someone who took his newfound strength and helped himself to heal from a catastrophic accident. He also said that what Marc had done was truly a miracle. Marc recalls, "A light bulb went off in my head right then and there. I was beginning to understand what I went through as I lay on the hard, cold floor of the warehouse. Out of something bad—being diabetic in my case—came something good. I had survived and would function as a whole person again. Thank you, diabetes!"

All of these stories of diabetes survivors just go to show you that, regardless of what you choose to accomplish in your lifetime, the choice to view yourself as empowered despite having diabetes is truly yours and yours alone. Once you make that proactive choice, you'll never want to go back to viewing yourself otherwise.

% 4 %

Maintain a Sense of Humor

Many long-living people with diabetes gave one of their top secrets as keeping a sense of humor about diabetes (and life) and laughing a lot. Research has shown that laughing lowers blood pressure, and in some people with diabetes, it may even lower their after-meal spikes in blood glucose. Having a greater ability to laugh in stressful situations may also lower your risk of developing heart disease. Could it be that laughter really is the best medicine?

Rich Humphreys is someone who has learned to laugh at every opportunity about diabetes and life in general. "You have to have a sense of humor with a chronic disease," he states. In the habit of turning lemons into lemonade (but not drinking it, of course, unless it's sugar free), he tells of a time when he pulled an elaborate trick after having surgery to fix a trigger finger caused by diabetes. He found a paper wasp nest that had been abandoned, and he flattened it and put it inside his bandage before he went to a doctor's appointment. It fell out when the nurse took off his bandage in the doctor's office, and she exclaimed, "I never heard of such a thing!"

Rich's return visit was scheduled for April Fools' Day, one of his most favorite days of the year, and he decided to take advantage of the spirit of the day when going back for his appointment. Beforehand, he made "scars" with rubber cement on his good (left) hand, let them dry, and then pinched them together. Then, he colored it pink with water colors and used a fine line permanent marker to draw on fake sutures. After wrapping it in an ace bandage, he headed off to the doctor's office with his 6-year-old son in tow, holding his son's hand with his right hand, the one that had really had the surgery. A different nurse came in to see him that day and then the doctor, who struggled for a while trying to figure out how to remove the fake sutures on Rich's good hand, until Rich finally wished him a happy April 1st and showed the befuddled doctor his other hand—the post-surgery one with the real sutures in it!

Mary Sue Rubin, who lives in Lutherville, Maryland, has had diabetes for almost 50 years (since the age of 9), and the first secret of her longevity that she listed was to have a sense of humor. "You have to have the ability to laugh at yourself," she says. Not surprisingly, Marc Blatstein, who owns his own consulting business, also feels that laughter is a key to success with diabetes. "I laugh and joke a lot . . . or sometimes I put on Motown music and sing along," he says. "I also do as many speaking engagements as I possibly can to help others smile and laugh with their diabetes. On the flip side, it helps me." He admits learning the power of laughter very early in life. "At the very young age of 10, I learned to laugh off problems and situations. I have always said, whether it be in front of an audience, on TV or radio, or just sitting with friends, 'Life handed me lemons with diabetes. So, I make lemonade!'"

Likewise, Jane Dohrmann expressed that for her, laughter is some of the best medicine she can find. She says, "Now, I have to admit that I use laughter at times when some people think it isn't appropriate. But I love to laugh, and it helps me get through everything!" One example she gave was when she recently underwent a heart catheterization and coronary artery stent placement. When her cardiologist asked her in all seriousness during the operation if she was doing well, she replied, "I am feeling just fine," but then she asked him, "How are *you* doing?"

Even Larry Verity advises that you find friends that understand your situation to help you make it through while keeping a sense of humor about it. Paul McGuigan agrees, and he adds that, "You have to find a way to get people to relax about diabetes—with a comment or a joke." Ron DeNunzio, a resident of Lancaster, Pennsylvania, who has had diabetes for 35 of his 46 years, recommends, "Look back at your diabetes and laugh at some of the situations you have had with it. At the moment, the situation might have been a low blood sugar, and you did something strange. Laughing makes diabetes fun." Although we fully understand what Ron is trying to say, we still doubt that there are many people who would use "diabetes" and "fun" in the same sentence!

✻ 5 ✻

Lose the Stress and the Guilt

A ny kind of stressor—either mental or physical—can cause a rise in both adrenaline and cortisol levels, which both decrease the action of insulin in your body and make blood sugars rise. Continuous or frequent psychological stress can make diabetes that much harder to control. A recent study involving stress management training for three months showed, however, that even people with diabetes can improve their glycemic control when they better learn to manage their stress. In another study, type 1 diabetic individuals with good glycemic control were found to manage their condition differently (e.g., doing more frequent home blood glucose tests) and use coping strategies that place greater emphasis on problem solving and being task-oriented. Similarly, a five-session, group stress management program in a "real-world" setting reduced stress and made diabetes control better in people with type 2 diabetes as well. Since having a chronic disease like diabetes can easily affect your psyche in negative ways, it's up to you to control the effect that stress has on your physical condition. Simple behaviors like conscious deep breathing, however, can help lower stress levels and improve your glucose control.

For some people, psychological stress is a conditioned response when it comes to medical checkups. For example, Carol Sessions experiences a lot of anxiety every time she goes to the doctor. A diabetes educator to whom she described her symptoms one time suggested that Carol might be experiencing a form of post-traumatic stress syndrome related to developing diabetes so early (at 3 years of age) and all of the medical visits, shots, and discomfort it entailed. Interestingly, a lot of people experience "white coat syndrome," meaning that they get stressed out at their doctors' offices. Because of this increased nervousness about the testing that will be done (and its possible results), it's not unusual for your blood pressure, for one, to be higher at your doctor's office than it normally is at home. It sometimes helps to have it measured a second time later in your visit if the reading is above normal the first time, or you can make arrangements to measure it yourself at home or somewhere else that doesn't evoke the same level of anxiety that can artificially raise your pressure. If you also experience emotional stress over getting your blood glucose measured during medical visits, make sure to measure it yourself before you visit your doctor so it also doesn't increase just from your upset related to the appointment.

Emotional stress, including depression, can also result from going through some of life's inevitable trials and tribulations. Stress and depressive disorders can seriously affect your ability to care for and control your health, often by decreasing your commitment to exercising regularly and/or following an appropriate diet. By way of example, Dan Spinazzola realizes that when he recently had to deal with a shoulder surgery that had gone badly, his brother's hospitalization and untimely death, and a lot of stress from his work, his blood sugars suffered. "All of it happening together really affected my blood sugars," he admits. "Things are better now, and I'm just starting to get back on target." Blondie Fram, who splits her time between Nashville, Tennessee, and Norfolk, Virginia, has been living with type 2 diabetes for more than 40 of her 93 years. She, too, notices that emotional stress really pushes her blood sugars up, so she tries not to let things bother her. She has had to go through treatments for breast cancer twice already, but she simply says, "I have learned to live with what I have to live with."

Anna Maria Gould finds that daily stress is one of biggest obstacles to good diabetes control. As a school counselor who has to respond to the needs of students and administrators alike, she finds the stress associated with her job to be unbelievably high at times, especially when it comes to deadlines. On days like those, she finds that she lets stress really affect her, and it hinders her diabetes control. "I try to work out as much as I can, but especially when my day is stressful. Working out relieves my stress, and it helps me have a good night's sleep." For Jane Dohrmann, learning to laugh at things has been a critical means to reduce her stress. Even Zach Barneis, a 23-year veteran of type 2 diabetes from Eshkolot, Israel, who at 68 years old says stress is one of his main barriers to good control. He recommends that everyone decrease stress as much as possible.

Sometimes, though, having a chronic disease like diabetes can afford you with a mind frame to worry less about things. "There have been times in my life," remarks Don Gifford, "when others are stressed out, and I can take a step back and choose not to stress, as most things are not as important as people make them out to be, and the majority are easier to deal with than having diabetes." Thus, controlling your mental state appears to come down simply to keeping things in perspective and making a decision not to let things stress you out too much or finding positive releases for those feelings. Although Karen Poenisch agrees that living a low-stress life is important, she thinks it's difficult to do with other people in it (especially kids). "I haven't noticed that big of an effect on my blood sugars, though," she says. "Maybe I'm stressed all the time and have just adapted to it!"

In addition to emotional issues, physical stress, be it from illness or lack of sleep, can also wreak havoc on blood sugars. "Try to get a good night's rest," says Vena Petrotta. She has a good point. Recent studies show that people who sleep too little (or even too much) have a greater chance of developing diabetes, likely due to the higher levels of cortisol elicited by not getting enough rest. Another of her secrets is to learn how to control emotions, especially anger and worrying. Bernadette McIntyre, a 49-year-old resident of Springfield, Pennsylvania, who has had diabetes since the age of 7 and a half, says, "I really think getting adequate rest promotes better health with diabetes. A lot of times when I do catch a virus or so, it is nearly always followed by a period of not getting enough rest and subsequent fatigue. I also believe this factor can be one in avoiding relapses in many diseases. My mom, being an RN herself, always stressed getting enough rest to me at an early age, and I thank her to this day for that." For Dr. Sheri, she finds that she can keep things in a better perspective and feel less anxious when she has had more rest. "It's when I'm physically tired that I tend to succumb to and experience the most mental stress," she says. Natalie Saunders agrees, stating unequivocally that "lack of sleep makes my blood sugars go up."

RELAX AND REDUCE YOUR STRESS FOR BETTER BLOOD GLUCOSE CONTROL

- Spend several minutes deep breathing—slowly inhaling and exhaling and visualizing the stress leaving your body.
- Sit quietly and imagine that you are in a calm, restful environment, such as at the beach, on a quiet hillside or mountain peak, or in the middle of the woods (whatever is most restful for you).
- Meditate by sitting quietly (preferably with your eyes closed), breathing slowly and deeply, and focusing all of your thoughts on one thing (an image in your mind, an object in the room, or a sound) for 10 to 20 minutes.
- Use progressive muscle relaxation, which is done by tensing an area of your body first and then fully relaxing it; try starting at your toes and working up your whole body.

- Listen to soothing music or relaxation tapes or CDs.
- Practice doing self-hypnosis, which is similar to meditation but usually uses positive affirmation (such as "I have a healthy body" or "I am in control of my diabetes") to manage stress and build self-confidence.
- Do yoga exercise and yoga deep breathing regularly.
- Go out for a brisk walk, or simply just get up and move around for a few minutes to get your blood flowing faster.

Similarly, feeling guilt over your diabetes and your glycemic control (or lack thereof) only contributes to both forms of stress. Natalie Saunders used to let her blood sugar swings bother her more than she does now. "I follow the book, but I'm not in excellent control," she says. "I'm just sensitive to when things upset me, and my blood sugar goes up and down. I just try to control my stress level."

For Chuck Eichten, his need to control his blood sugars has sometimes bordered on being obsessive. He says, "Every glucose reading can seem like a personal test. You want to know, did you pass or fail? If it's not what you thought it should be, you think you must have done something wrong." In more recent years, he has learned to relax a bit more and not feel so guilty when his sugars go a little bit out of his expected range. Jessica Ching from San Diego, California, has a similar outlook. She says, "You have to accept that you'll never have full control over your diabetes." Although she admits to being in denial for the first 12 years she had diabetes (she was diagnosed in 1979 when she was 16), she took control of her life and her diabetes when she went on an insulin pump back in 1991. "Don't let it get to you," she advises, "or it will destroy you. Just accept your diabetes and do what works for you. If you want to have chocolate and sweets every day, find out how to integrate it into your life."

Dan Spinazzola admits to not being a model person with diabetes, although he tries hard. He feels guilty about going off his diet and eating some cookies—which he spent his whole life eating until he was diagnosed with diabetes at the age of 49—but his old habits have died hard. "I'll eat too many and then feel guilty," he says, "but then my denial kicks in, along with my rationalizations. For me, everything leads to a cookie." An occasional slip should not be a reason to throw in the towel, though. "Exceptions to your diet are okay, as long as they're not routine," Patty Schaeffer reminds us.

Guilt comes from many potential situations, sometimes from knowing you could take better care of yourself, but also from feeling like you're letting other people down because of your diabetes. Marc Blatstein shares the guilt he felt about his diabetes diagnosis at the age of 10: "I looked up in awe at my parents crying as they told me I had diabetes. I wasn't upset about the diagnosis—I was upset because I had so upset them. I carried that guilt around for many years." Feeling guilty almost never helps improve your diabetes control, though, and guilt is an emotion better left traded in for a positive attitude and a better mental outlook.

Jim Turner, a 55-year-old comedian and actor living in Los Angeles, California, diagnosed with diabetes almost 38 years ago, finds that talking to other people with diabetes, hearing their stories, and sharing yours with them helps. "Any guilt or shame you feel is less when you share it with others," he advises. "It really helps me—and a lot of other people, too."

Another reason to try to enhance and uplift your mood is the poorly understood mind-body connection. Physical health and mental health are undeniably interrelated, and each affects the other. Therefore, your physical well-being often can't be improved if your psychological problems haven't been adequately addressed. The best advice is to learn how to lower your levels of stress and feelings of guilt to help you live longer and better with your diabetes.

❧ 6 ❧

Reach for the Stars

A vital part of living well with diabetes is to set goals, pursue your dreams, and make them a reality, in spite of living with a chronic disease. An inspiring example of such goal setting took place when Patricia La France-Wolf lost her sight due to diabetic eye problems over 30 years ago. Instead of sitting around and feeling sorry for herself (okay, she did that for a few days), she decided to go back to school and get a master's degree in rehabilitation counseling. Since finishing her degree, she has taught other blind individuals for years how to live well despite their disability, including teaching blind people with diabetes how to use talking blood glucose meters and how to deal with the emotional issues associated with diabetes and its complications. "Nothing stays good all the time," she says, "but nothing stays bad all the time either. You have to persevere even when things aren't going good."

Rich Humphreys, now 65 years old, had a goal to go around the world by the time he was 33. In reaching his goal, he crossed Europe, worked for eight weeks in Israel, flew to Anchorage and hitchhiked down the Alaskan coast, bicycled to Oregon, dipped his bike into the Pacific Ocean, and then biked back to his home in Pennsylvania—completing the last leg of his journey (going across the United States) in just forty-five days. What was most amazing was that he did all of it by himself *and* without having a blood glucose meter. He experienced a few bad lows along the way, but he just kept going until he accomplished his goal.

For Jim Turner, diabetes was just another obstacle to be overcome. From early on in his diabetic life, he was determined to do "whatever," and he set goals to accomplish the things he wanted to do. For example, he decided to go on a three-month bike trip across Europe in 1973 when he was just 21 years old. He started out on the trip with another friend, but he had to continue on alone after his traveling companion was injured by being hit by a car. "I was riding across Italy and Germany for a month all alone—without knowing what my blood sugar was," he recalls. "The trip gave me the feeling that I could do it, no matter what 'it' is."

Some individuals have set athletic goals, many resulting in Olympic medals (see more on these athletes in Secret 29). One of the longer-living athletes who set early goals and attained them, though, is Doug Burns from Mississippi, who has lived with diabetes for more 36 years since the age of 7. Finally winning the title of "Mr. Natural Universe" in 2006 for his drug-free bodybuilding, he realized one of his biggest athletic goals by becoming the first ever such title winner with type 1 diabetes. As a youngster with diabetes before blood glucose meters were available, his diabetes control was poor, and he was unable to participate in sports, at least until he began lifting weights to become stronger. After setting state, regional, and American records in drug-free power lifting and winning six power-lifting championships, he turned to bodybuilding competitions, eventually winning titles for "Mr. Southern States," "Mr. California," and "Mr. USA" just a couple of years ago, before his recent crowning with the ultimate "Mr. Universe" title.

When another athlete, Bill King of Aston, Pennsylvania, was diagnosed at the age of 24, he was already a marathon runner. His body had been stressed by a combination of overtraining (running excessive mileage), working two jobs, going to school, getting over a romantic breakup, and overcoming a viral infection when he was diagnosed with diabetes over 23 years ago. At the time that his doctor told him the diagnosis, his first thought was just that he needed to know what to do about it so he could get back to running. To this day, he still credits his goal to continue running (which he has done, running seventeen marathons since that time) for his continuing good health.

Your goals don't have to be monumental; for example, they can simply revolve around having good health and living long with diabetes. To this end, Bob Cleveland recommends, "You have to be cautious about your diet and keep a constant check on your blood glucose levels." His goals throughout his lifetime have mainly revolved around keeping the best control over his diabetes that he could by using whatever management tools were available to him, practices that have served him well over his very long and exceedingly healthy lifetime with diabetes. Although Jane Dohrmann has only lived half as long as Bob has with diabetes, she agrees that finding the determination to achieve your goals, whatever they may be, is important for anyone with a chronic disease like diabetes.

For James "Jim" Arthur, a resident of Lake Wylie, South Carolina, who has been living with diabetes for 64 of his 74 years, his goal was also to survive long and well with diabetes, which he has done so far. When he was about 13 or 14, he remembers being at his best friend's house and overhearing a comment that made him set that goal. His best friend's mother, Mrs. Young, was talking to a friend of hers and was unaware that Jim had come into the house and could hear them. From the next room, he heard her say, "It's really too bad about James. It'll be a miracle if he makes it to 45." He took it as a personal challenge to prove her wrong. Although Mrs. Young has long since died herself. Jim remarks, "Mrs. Young would be surprised that I've almost made it to 75 already." Thirty years (and counting) past his predicted demise. Jim appeared to have exceeded even his own expectations.

If having strong goals or motivating factors is what is going to help you live long and well with diabetes as well, then we're all for them! So, go ahead and reach for the stars, and you may just get lucky. If you only end up on the moon, at least you will know that you gave it your all, and working toward your goal likely improved the quality of your life along the way.

GERALD CLEVELAND, AGE 91, LIVING WITH TYPE 1 DIABETES FOR 75 YEARS

A life-time resident of the Syracuse, New York, area, Gerald Cleveland has had a lifetime of not quite measuring up—at least until now. As salutatorian (the second-ranking person in a graduating class after the valedictorian) of his high school's graduating class, his collegiate program in education, and his master's degree, he good-heartedly complains that he was "always coming in second." In fact, even his brother Bob has had diabetes for 7 years longer, making Gerald second in line when it comes to longevity with the disease in his family. However, he's first in line when it comes to being the oldest individual living with diabetes for most of his lifetime (he's a year older than Gladys Dull), and when he makes it to his 100th birthday (as he plans to do), he'll be the first one to achieve that honor with type 1 diabetes as well. (Gerald's profile in this book is also coming before his brother Bob's, so it's about time that he accepts that he's finally moving to the front of the line in some things.)

For the rest of us who have not had to live with diabetes nearly as long as Gerald, it's hard to conceive of having to take insulin doses that filled a whole syringe just to cover one meal, using a needle that had to be sharpened on a whetstone and felt like a knitting needle going in, or going for at least the first 50 years of having diabetes without the benefit of a blood glucose meter. Being the second child in his family to get diabetes (after brother Bob) was not a good place in line either, as he had already seen Bob having to suffer through diabetes treatments for 7 years. He took it on with a positive attitude, though, coming up with innovative ways to control diabetes with the tools he had available. For instance, he even rigged up a quart pot with holes to put test tubes in (instead of holding them over a Bunsen burner) so that he and his brother could test the sugar in their urine more easily back in the early days.

Labeled "an archeological find" by his doctor, this long-living brother attributes his longevity with diabetes to being active (walking long distances most of his life), being vigilant about his diet, and having faith that the best things in life always lie ahead. His vigilance about his diabetes control is readily apparent, though. One of his first diabetes doctors at the University Hospital at Syracuse gave him a menu of what he should eat to control his diabetes, and to this day, he still has it posted on the door of his kitchen. He describes controlling diabetes as similar to "walking on a tightrope that's swinging in the air," but admits to having developed a better sense than most about the effect of carbs in general and different portion sizes on his blood sugars. He gets frustrated by other people's misconceptions about food, such as when they mistakenly believe that "sugar-free" desserts will not have any effect on their blood glucose levels (since they still usually contain large amounts of carbs).

Gerald admits, "I have had a wonderful blessing of longevity and being a useful person," a role that he still fills to this day. He had a long career in education, serving first as a secondary school teacher of social studies, choosing later to become the first male elementary teacher in Syracuse and then the principal of an elementary junior high, earning his doctorate in education (EdD) while working as assistant superintendent of their public school system 27 years, and finally serving as superintendent for one before his retirement. He was a member of the team that founded the public TV station there, along with Junior Achievement, and he also served as an elder at his local Presbyterian Church for 70 years and worked for the Syracuse Rescue Mission (serving the homeless and hurting of Central New York) for many years. He has recently been honored as an outstanding alumnus of Syracuse University, as well as being recognized by the Joslin Diabetes Center and Lilly Pharmaceuticals for his longevity with diabetes. He even donates his time at the Nottingham Center, where he currently lives in Jamesville, New York, acting as a consultant and advisor to help other residents learn how to live better with diabetes.

His life has also been blessed with a sixty-two-year marriage (that ended in 2002 with his wife Mildred's passing), two children, five grandchildren, and five great-grandchildren to date. His wife was vigilant about checking to see if his blood sugars were low at night and generally looking out for him (not that he needed too much help). To this day, his daughter continues to check in on him frequently, calling him three times daily to make certain that his blood sugars are not too low. Regardless of any physical ailments he has had related to his diabetes (such as the loss of two toes on his right foot), he has always kept a positive outlook. He truly believes that there are angels all around him—looking out for him—because whenever he has found himself having difficulty with his diabetes, someone or something has been there to help him.

When it comes to being a diabetes celebrity, he admits feeling a bit uncomfortable. "I feel like a very ordinary guy, but then there's this other person that everyone looks up to that hardly feels like me—the one who's an inspiration to so many people living with diabetes. I'm just afraid of letting them down somehow." Not much chance of that, Gerald!

ROBERT "BOB" CLEVELAND, AGE 87, LIVING WITH TYPE 1 DIABETES FOR 82 YEARS

Not to be outdone by his older brother (the oldest living person with diabetes most of his life), Bob Cleveland is believed to be the person who has lived the longest with type 1 diabetes to date after Gladys Dull (who only beats him by less than a year)—since being diagnosed in 1925, shortly after insulin became commercially available. Certainly, you can attribute a part of his successful life span to inheriting good genes, but there is much more to his longevity than that. Even though he was only 5 when he was diagnosed with diabetes, more than four-fifths of a century ago, Bob still remembers the day he went into the hospital for diabetes. "I thought I was going to the hospital to die," he admits. Although he had wasted away to skin and bones, they still initially put him on a "starvation diet" to control his blood sugars, a standard treatment in the pre-insulin era. Luckily for him, insulin had just been discovered in 1921 and was available to treat him. Once the doctors finally got his insulin doses adjusted and were able to put him on a diet to gain some of the weight back, he was sent home.

His early years with diabetes were particularly challenging. He remembers things being "touch and go" for a time, with his mother pulling him out of diabetic comas caused by low blood sugars, while trying to take care of his three siblings. "There was no way to really test for blood sugar levels back then, so everything was strictly a guess," he recalls. He and his mother realized the positive effects of exercise early on, though, even while relying on ineffective and inaccurate urine testing methods. "I was taking lots of insulin, but Mom would cut back on my doses when I exercised a lot. She could tell by testing my urine. If there was no sugar in it, she cut back my dose." (To her credit, her methods of insulin adjustment were well ahead of the standard medical practice at the time.) To this day, he is still an avid cyclist, often riding twenty miles or more outdoors on any given day, even though he can't walk nearly as far as he used to due to weakness in his leg muscles. When he rides, he has found that he can sometimes go all day without taking any insulin other than his normal dose of long-acting basal insulin (Lantus), and yet his blood sugars stay good all day long.

Bob is proud of having diabetes and likes to help anyone he can, but in his earlier years, he didn't feel free to talk about it. In fact, for most of his life, he says that "diabetes was a "disease that nobody talked about." He found out the hard way that potential employers were often less than enamored with his diabetic state. He majored in accounting in college, but lost several jobs after admitting on the application form that he had diabetes. As a result, he found himself having to lie about his physical condition in order to get hired. "After I heard several times, 'we'll call you if and when there's an opening . . . ,' I stopped admitting that I have diabetes. I finally got in as an accountant with General Motors in Syracuse, but I had to lie about my disease." Diabetes couldn't have been too much of an impediment, since he went on to have a long and productive career in his chosen field, eventually becoming the supervisor of GM's general accounting section there for many years.

Admittedly, sitting behind a desk all day with ledgers and a telephone is part of the reason why he has been so active in the rest of his life. "After sitting there all day, when I left my office, I just wanted to be outside as much as I could." He attributes his continuing good health to a combination of getting plenty of exercise, being cautious about his diet, keeping a constant check on his blood sugars, and having a loving and supportive spouse (he has been married almost six decades to his wife Ruth). His longevity and good health have been acknowledged, along with brother Gerald's, by both the Joslin Diabetes Center and Lilly Pharmaceutical Company, who put up a monument to the brothers in Indianapolis, Indiana, a couple of years ago. "I really feel blessed living as long as I have. Even doctors at the Joslin Diabetes Center have never talked to anyone who's had diabetes as long as I have." Maybe Bob's goal should be to become the first person in the history of diabetes to have it for a full century. If anyone can do it, he can!

PART TWO

Knowledge Secrets

Be Your Own Best Advocate

Ultimately, you're in charge of your own diabetes, so the best thing you can do is to take responsibility for it and become your own diabetes advocate. Empower yourself by using any knowledge you have acquired to seek out better ways to control your diabetes. Some people may be in great denial about their health, or they may just not want to hear about what they have to do or what they're doing wrong. In the case of diabetes, ignorance is not bliss, though. What you ignore or don't treat properly can and likely will come back to haunt you in the form of one health problem or another. Patricia La France-Wolf recognizes the importance of taking responsibility, and she teaches this concept to others in diabetes education classes for the blind. "You have to be responsible for your own care," she asserts. Peter Gariti agrees, saying, "You have to have self-discipline."

Dolores "Dee" Brehm, a 58-year survivor of diabetes from McClain, Virginia, developed the condition during her sophomore year at Eastern Michigan University at the age of 19. From the start, she had to take complete responsibility for her own diabetes management. "My parents never even asked me about it," she remembers. Her biggest obstacle to taking charge of her condition was that she got very little education about what to do when she was diagnosed in 1949. "They gave me a sheet of what to eat and what not to eat, but no counseling and few recommendations." Much to her credit, she has gained a vast knowledge of diabetes since that time. Such information is abundant nowadays, and you can use it to take responsibility for your diabetes care from the start.

The reality is that many people have gone through periods of their lives when they chose to ignore their diabetes, especially when there was less information available about diabetes around and fewer tools with which to control it. Even Don Gifford went through a period of worse control during his teens and 20s when he was a bit rebellious and chose to run high instead of risking getting low. Marc Blatstein had a similar period. He says, "Throughout my teenage years, I treated my diabetes as if it just wasn't a problem and that everything would fix itself. How wrong I was!"

Ron DeNunzio rebelled against controlling his diabetes on many occasions when he was younger. "I would eat candy every chance I had, although I would drink diet soda (Tab). Sometime in the mid-1980s I went to a diabetic doctor, and I still did not listen. I got a blood glucose meter that I never used." Unfortunately, Ron ended up learning the hard way that good control from the start of your diabetes and diligence about staying in control is important in preventing complications later on, as most of the long-time survivors with diabetes have discovered. Ron now lists one of the secrets of longevity as "Become your advocate for your diabetes."

Dr. Steve remembers when he worked at a (nondiabetic) boys' camp in Los Angeles every summer and almost every weekend during the rest of the school year as a camp aid, cook, and counselor. Every week they had a contest called, for lack of a better name, "The Pissing Contest," the goal of which was to see who could urinate for the longest period of time. He recalls, "We took this event seriously, even using a stopwatch that measured to 1/100th of a second. During competition, you had to have one continuous stream, done with your hands behind your back so you couldn't do any weird manipulations to increase your time. Well, I remember winning week after week after week, and I still hold the camp record to this day. Just try urinating continuously for one minute and fifteen seconds straight without stopping!" The not-so-funny thing about this story is that his diabetes was horribly out of control, resulting in excessive thirst and urination.

"I was not a rebellious teenager who purposely went out of control for attention," Dr. Steve says. "It took me several years to realize that I should do something about the fact that I was probably not doing well, despite my doctor's repeated comments about my 'doing fine.' Home glucose monitors and the hemoglobin A1c test (a blood measure of overall blood glucose control over the previous two to three months) were not invented at that time, so I truly did not know that I was doing harm to my body. I simply was never told what my goals of control should be and why it was so important in a way that I understood at the time." He has certainly gone out of his way to make up for his early lack of knowledge (and diabetes control) since then, though.

Some individuals who got diabetes really early in life were forced to rely on their parents to gather the information for them, at least initially. Karen Poenisch, who was 8 years old at the time of her diagnosis, remembers that she and her family were given no real information about diet. Her mother sought out help, locating a dietitian living in her grandmother's neighborhood, and from her they got the dietary advice to cut out sugar and watch fat intake. Since that time, Karen herself has become a diabetes educator, a role she has filled for the past 28 years, helping people with diabetes interested in using insulin pumps and, most recently, continuous glucose-monitoring devices. If you are a parent of a child with either type of diabetes, it's good to know that you have a wealth of information available to you now that you can access and pass on to your son or daughter in the near future.

The sooner you realize that your health is up to you and take responsibility for your own care, though, the better your health is likely to be in the long run. Bill King, who interacts with a lot of people with diabetes and health-care professionals in his job, says, "You shouldn't leave all your diabetes care to your health-care team. We're living in a time now when the health-care industry is overwhelmed, and there's less time for anyone to spend with his or her doctor." He believes that diabetes is the tsunami of the health-care system, and anyone aware of the growing epidemic of diabetes is likely to agree (including both of us). "You have to get some of the information on your own," Bill advises. "If you have an outdated glucose meter, get yourself a newer one. Consider going on a pump if you use insulin. Don't depend on your doctor to make those decisions for you."

Dr. Steve is the ultimate cheerleader in diabetes self-advocacy. He is founder and director of Taking Control of Your Diabetes (TCOYD), a national not-for-profit organization whose mission is the following: "To educate and motivate people with diabetes, and their loved ones, to take a more active role in their condition in order to live healthier, happier, and more productive lives." He always encourages people to learn how to take control of their diabetes and become empowered and knowledgeable enough to advocate for their own best health-care interests, regardless of their age or type of diabetes. He says, "Knowing about the latest advances in diabetes care and being able to get them is key to living well with diabetes—and it's an essential part of being your own best advocate."

❧ 8 ❧

Learn All You Can about Diabetes

K nowledge is power. Everyone agrees that a critical secret of
diabetes longevity is to learn as much as you can about your
disease. Many survivors recommend reading anything and everything you can about diabetes and using the information you learn
to motivate yourself to better control your condition. Controlling
diabetes is only one aspect of having a healthy body for a lifetime,
although it is a critical one for anyone living with it.

When he was diagnosed with type 2 diabetes, Zach Barneis
bought the American Diabetes Association's series of books on
diabetes and followed a very strict diet by counting carbohydrates. He recalls, "Everything was self-taught and disciplined,
with periodic visits to an endocrinologist." He believes that a key
to longevity is to know as much about diabetes as possible, what
its effects on your body can be, and your general health situation.
"In this respect," he says, "it is much easier today because of the
wealth of information available on the Internet, the number of
support/discussion groups, and mailing lists." Similarly, Rabbi
Meisels recommends reading up on diabetes and not just relying
on what you're being told.

In teaching diabetes education classes to the blind, Patricia La
France-Wolf came up with a list of five things that she feels are
most important to effective diabetes control, regardless of the
type: diet, responsibility, exercise, attitude, and medicine. "Education is extremely important," she says. "Many newly diagnosed
people with type 2 diabetes still don't get enough education nowadays. You can't just tell people to eat lots of fruits and veggies." The

more specific the advice is with regard to diet, exercise, and medications, she feels the easier it is for people to follow.

Larry Verity would have to agree that education makes all the difference for many people. He says, "One of the best things that happened to me when I was diagnosed over 30 years ago was what the nurse said to me. She warned me that we don't know a lot about diabetes, but that I should read as much as possible to learn more." To this day, he continues to seek out more knowledge about diabetes even though he has amassed a large amount of information already. Likewise, Karen Poenisch agrees that education is very important (as she should, since she's a diabetes educator). She believes that knowing how insulin works and when it peaks are crucial. "You don't want to exercise during the peak of your insulin," she says. Another believer in education, Judy Tripathi, who works as a dietitian at Integrated Diabetes Services in Wynnewood, Pennsylvania, feels that working around people who are so knowledgeable about diabetes and being exposed to so many diabetes resources has changed her life. "I try my best to instill knowledge and inspiration into my patients," she says, and she lets all of it rub off onto herself, too. Mary Sue Rubin thinks that diabetes education is important, but so is general information about living a healthy life (with or without diabetes).

"Education is so important—I feel so strongly about it," says Carolyn Balcom. "I never stop learning about diabetes, and I will probably never stop. I want to learn all I can about how to take care of myself." She adds that being a nurse has helped her, as well as having some basic information to start with. "In nursing school, the instructors emphasized that if a person followed the rules, the chances of complications were much less likely—and I believed this from the beginning, both as a nurse and someone with diabetes." Jane Dohrmann agrees. "I'm a proverbial sponge and want to know whatever I can about whatever is out there that can help me be a healthier person with diabetes," she says.

Natalie Saunders also has tried to find as much information as she could over 36 years with diabetes, going several times to visit the Joslin Clinic in Boston while on her quest. "Knowledge is good," she affirms. "You have to talk to people, ask questions, find out what you can, read up on diabetes. I've also gotten lots of information from my diabetes educator lately." Chuck Eichten also feels strongly that education is important for understanding diabetes conceptually. "For me, learning about diabetes means understanding it to the best of my ability so that I really know what's going on with my body," he says. "I don't want to just be doing what I was told to do; I want to be able to think it through to make the right decisions for myself."

Ron DeNunzio thinks the best education comes from other people who have diabetes, particularly those who are health-care professionals, like Dr. Steve. Even Paul McGuigan found that he had a passion to learn about diabetes, which led him to switch from being a house painter and decorator to pursue a degree in nursing after his diabetes diagnosis at the age of 24. He says, "My current job has made it easier to deal with my own diabetes because of the knowledge base I have access to. I have had lots of support from people who understand diabetes, like endocrinologists at work and others." He notes that having access to supplies and equipment and lab tests at work also has helped, although he did get diabetes right around the time that blood glucose meters were coming out, so he has had access to one most of his diabetic life. Also in agreement, Bill King says that one of his secrets of living well with diabetes and having no complications to date is that he is surrounded by people with diabetes at his workplace. "I see the successful cases," he says, "and seeing that has put me on an insatiable quest for more knowledge. A willingness to try new things is important, too."

Patty Schaeffer also recommends staying abreast of what's going on in the diabetes world, which has really taken off during the last two decades since the wide availability of blood glucose meters in the 1980s. "Join the American Diabetes Association, and read their magazines," she advises. You can also get print materials from many other sources, as well as online access (see Looking for More Diabetes Information? for places to look). In fact, there is so much information available about diabetes nowadays that you'd have to work hard to avoid being exposed to any of it. For instance, if you just search the keywords "diabetes care" on Google, you get over 1.5 million hits! Then there's the blossoming number of diabetes blogs, forums, e-mail newsletters, and Web chats. You could spend all your days searching the Net and likely never run out of things to read about diabetes. Just be careful about the source, and make sure it's a reputable one. Also, check with your diabetes health-care provider before making changes to your diabetes medication or regimen that you found out about using online resources.

LOOKING FOR MORE DIABETES INFORMATION? HERE'S A SHORT LIST OF PLACES TO SEARCH

Diabetes Magazines (Print and Online Access or Subscription Information)

Countdown and Countdown for Kids (Juvenile Diabetes Research Foundation: www.jdrf.org; 800-533-CURE [2873]; info@jdrf.org)

Diabetes Forecast (American Diabetes Association: www.diabetes.org; 800-DIABETES, or 800-342-2383; AskADA@diabetes.org)

Diabetes Health; online: www.diabeteshealth.com (and e-newsletters); 800-488-8468

Diabetes Self-Management; online: www.diabetesselfmanagement.com (and e-newsletters); 800-234-0923; webeditor@diabetes-self-mgmt.com

Diabetic Cooking; online: www/diabeticcooking.com; 800-777-5582

Diabetic Gourmet; online: www.diabeticgourmet.com

Diabetic Living (Better Homes and Gardens: www.bhg.com)

Voice of the Diabetic (National Federation of the Blind); online: www.nfb.org/nfb/Voice_of_the_Diabetic.asp (free publication print or online)

Additional Web Resources

American Diabetes Association: www.diabetes.org (articles, bookstore, podcasts)

CDC Division of Diabetes Translation: www.cdc.gov/diabetes/pubs/general.htm

Children with Diabetes: www.childrenwithdiabetes.com (for parents and kids)

David Mendosa—A Writer on the Web: www.mendosa.com (extensive links to Web sites, chat rooms, support groups, newsletters, blogs, publications, and more)

Diabetes Sports and Wellness Foundation: www.dswf.org (type 1 and exercise)

Diabetes Exercise & Sports Association (DESA): www.diabetes-exercise.org

Diabetes In Control: www.diabetesincontrol.com (weekly research updates)

Diabetes Institutes Foundation: www.dif.org (INGAP research and information)

Diabetes Mine: www.diabetesmine.org (Amy Tenderich's educational site and blog)

Diabetes Monitor: www.diabetesmonitor.com (and companion diabetes.blog.com)

dLife—For Your Diabetes Life: www.dlife.com (information and TV show)

Dr. Sheri Colberg's Web site: www.shericolberg.com (exercise information, books, articles, forum, and more)

Friends with Diabetes: www.friendswithdiabetes.org (Judaism-specific information)

Juvenile Diabetes Research Foundation: www.jdrf.org (newsletters)

National Diabetes Education Program: www.ndep.nih.gov (patient resources)

National Diabetes Information Clearinghouse: diabetes.niddk.nih.gov (basic diabetes information, statistics, etc.)

Taking Control of Your Diabetes (TCOYD): www.tcoyd.org (newsletters, TV show, articles, and Dr. Steve's columns on site)

The Diabetes Mall: www.diabetesnet.com (diabetic supplies and information)

One of Dr. Steve's main barriers to controlling his diabetes early on was that he had received a limited education when he was diagnosed in 1970. Getting diabetes at 15, he would have been old enough to absorb what he needed to know to take care of himself, but he instead was put in a diabetes education class at Kaiser Permanente (a health maintenance organization) with 39 overweight type 2s that taught him little. He remembers learning only that ketchup has sugar (and was therefore forbidden) and wondering what he was going to put on his French fries from then on. The doctor who taught him about urine testing and put him on one shot of NPH (Humulin N) and Regular insulin a day was a big, fat guy who smoked—not quite the healthy role model Dr. Steve was looking for. He blames his lack of education about how to control his blood sugars for his early onset of complications: diabetic retinopathy in 1981 after only 11 years with diabetes. He advises everyone, "Be as educated as possible. It's your diabetes, and knowledge is key to living well with it."

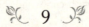

9

Share Your Wealth of Knowledge

Once you learn about more about diabetes and how to control it, everyone wins when you choose to share your knowledge with others. What can you do to share the wisdom that comes from your personal (and sometimes professional) experiences? You can get involved as a diabetes camp counselor, do diabetes-related volunteer work, and be a role model for kids and other people with diabetes. A good example of these sorts of sharing activities is Marc Blatstein, who has taught and counseled thousands of people with diabetes over the past two decades, saying that doing so helped him, too. He never hesitates to talk about his diabetes or the issues he has had living with it. Studies have shown that this type of positive support from people like Marc also fosters the desire for adolescents with diabetes at summer camps and others to take better care of themselves, which in turn improves their health and their quality of life.

Rich Humphreys also stresses the importance of being a positive role model for others with diabetes, particularly kids. He should know, since he has directed a camp for diabetic kids for more than twenty years near Cleveland, Ohio, called Camp Ho Mita Koda. Just recently, he purposefully made the 380-mile walk from the camp in Ohio to his home in southern Lancaster County, Pennsylvania, and his five-week journey made quite a statement to the kids attending the camp who knew of his endeavor. Carol Sessions has additionally experienced the benefits of learning and sharing your knowledge in a summer camp setting. As a kid, she attended a long-standing diabetes camp in the California mountains at Bearskin Meadows, where diabetic kids rough it by sleeping outside on platforms during camp. (Even in the summer, it can be a cold experience!) She returned to camp as a counselor-in-training and shared a lot of her experience with younger campers, even though she went to camp way before blood glucose meters were available. For Marialice Kern, working as a camp counselor at Bearskin Meadows Camp for diabetic kids right after she was diagnosed at the age of 19 not only allowed her to learn everything she needed to know, but also enabled her to turn right around and share her newfound knowledge with younger kids at camp.

Jane Dohrmann has found another outlet to help others by

volunteering for and joining diabetes-related organizations. "I am a volunteer for the Juvenile Diabetes Research Foundation (JDRF), and I have been a member of the ADA (American Diabetes Association) since I was a young child," she reports. More recently, she was asked to help out online at www.insulinpumpers.com. "It makes me feel like I'm doing something positive for others with diabetes like my first diabetic friend did for me so many years ago." Similarly, Julie Krupnick, who lives in Virginia Beach and has had diabetes for 28 years, started volunteering frequently for her local chapter of the ADA. Ron DeNunzio has also gotten heavily involved in both the ADA and diabetic summer camps, which he finds to be a great outlet for sharing the knowledge he has gained about avoiding diabetic complications through his own difficult experiences. Although there are many worthy local, regional, and national groups supporting diabetes research and educational programs for which you can volunteer your time, the major ones (i.e., the ADA and JDRF) are given in the box that follows this section.

INTERESTED IN VOLUNTEERING YOUR TIME FOR DIABETES? TRY THESE GROUPS AND SOME OF THEIR FUNDRAISING AND OTHER EVENTS FIRST

American Diabetes Association:

Volunteering: www.diabetes.org/support-the-cause/volunteer-with-us.jsp; 800-DIABETES, or 800-342-2383

Diabetes Camps (local camps listed at www.diabetes.org/communityprograms-and-localevents/diabetescamps/nationwide.jsp; on the Children with Diabetes Web site found at www.childrenwithdiabetes.com/camps; or at Diabetes Education & Camping Association at www.diabetescamps.org)

Local Events: www.diabetes.org/communityprograms-and-localevents.jsp

America's Walk for Diabetes (annual fundraising walk in October/November by region)

Tour de Cure (annual spring 30- to 100-mile cycling event in more than 80 cities to benefit the ADA)

Diabetes EXPO (interactive events in U.S. cities to provide access to health-care providers, educators, exhibitors, and health screenings)

Community Campaign for Diabetes (donation campaign: www.diabetes.org/support-the-cause/community-campaign.jsp)

Juvenile Diabetes Research Foundation:

Volunteering: www.jdrf.org; 800-533-CURE (2873); info@jdrf.org

Online Diabetes Support Team (emotional and educational support for newly diagnosed type 1 families provided by parents who've "been there")

Children's Congress (biannual event when children with diabetes from all states come to Washington, D.C., together to advocate for a cure for diabetes)

Promise to Remember Me Campaign (annual pilgrimage to Washington, D.C., to educate members congress about the need for research for a cure for diabetes)

Local Events:

Walk to Cure Diabetes (family-friendly fundraising walks held in over 200 cites nationwide; walk.jdrf.org; 888-533-WALK)

Ride to Cure Diabetes (cycling fundraising events at more than five locations; ride.jdrf.org)

Many other people with diabetes are drawn to health professions and end up specializing in diabetes care. Both of the authors of this book are good examples. Dr. Steve is a well-respected endocrinologist who mainly treats people with diabetes, and his calling to help others has been so profound that he does it large-scale now through more than a dozen TCOYD conferences and health fairs annually, a new TCOYD TV show on MD-TV, local seminars given in San Diego, and a TCOYD quarterly newsletter. Dr. Sheri was also drawn to the study of exercise physiology initially because it was the only thing that made her feel better when she was young (and already diagnosed with diabetes). Although her doctoral research was on glucose metabolism in smokers (hey, you go with whatever funding your professor has at the time), all of her subsequent research to this day has focused on diabetes control and prevention with exercise. Similarly, two of the interviewees for this book, Marialice Kern and Larry Verity, have doctoral degrees in exercise physiology and an interest in diabetes research as well, although both of them developed diabetes in their late teens or early adulthood. We also interviewed many nurses, diabetes educators, dietitians, and other diabetes health-care providers who have diabetes themselves.

10

Understand Possible Diabetes Complications

Wouldn't it be easier to bury your head in the sand and avoid thinking about all of the more common potential health consequences of diabetes? Well, it might be, but only until you started experiencing one and had to deal with it, particularly as many of them are now preventable with effective use of home blood glucose meters that finally hit the market in the 1980s. Unfortunately, though, complications are still possible (even if you know about them) and a reality for many people living with diabetes. The best thing you can do, then, is to strive to understand what causes them, what symptoms to look out for, and how to prevent yourself from getting them in the first place.

Studies leave no doubt that elevated blood sugar levels over time can potentially be very damaging to your eyes, kidneys, and nerves. By now, practically all of us have been counseled about the possibility of developing the three "opathies": retinopathy (diabetic eye disease), nephropathy (kidney disease), and neuropathy (nerve damage), some of the better known and more common complications associated with type 1 and type 2 diabetes. In fact, poorly controlled diabetes is the leading cause of new cases of blindness among adults. Proliferative diabetic retinopathy (a severe form of diabetic eye disease that can cause hemorrhaging into the eye, vision loss, and retinal detachment) itself causes tens of thousands of new cases of blindness each year, only some of which are reversible with a vitrectomy (removal and replacement of the fluid inside the eye). In addition, diabetes can cause six other types of eye disease that can negatively impact your vision, such as glaucoma, cataracts, macular degeneration, and neuropathy of the optic or eye muscle nerves.

Of the more than fifty people that we interviewed for this book, two-thirds of them with diabetes between 40 and 83 years, just over twenty to date, have developed some level of retinopathy, and nine have had cataract surgery. One thing to keep in mind, though, is that the longer-living people with diabetes we interviewed went for many years without the benefit of knowing what their blood sugars were (or necessarily controlling them well), which luckily no longer is as common, since blood glucose meters are inexpensive and widely available. In current times, the incidence of eye complications is dropping, and some preventive treatments for retinopathy are also in the works, which may serve to prevent it altogether in most individuals.

Your kidneys can be similarly negatively affected by diabetes, making it the leading cause of new cases of kidney disease that have to be treated by dialysis and ultimately kidney transplants. Of the people interviewed, although six had been diagnosed with signs of nephropathy, none has progressed to the point of needing dialysis. In many cases, progression of kidney disease can be put on hold or delayed considerably with the use of certain medications that protect kidney function, as Dr. Steve has done for almost two decades already.

Traditionally, 60 to 70 percent of diabetic individuals also experience mild to severe nerve damage, symptoms of which include impaired sensation (numbness) or shooting pains (painful neuropathy) in feet or hands, gastroparesis (slowing of the digestion of food), orthostatic hypertension (severe dizziness when standing up), and even erectile dysfunction in men and decreased sexual function in women. A lower percentage of our interviewees (about 30 percent) are currently dealing with any type of neuropathy, though, and only four have been experiencing severe problems with gastroparesis (symptoms like nausea, vomiting, bloating, abdominal pain, heartburn, and alternating diarrhea and constipation). Diabetic ulcers, often related to nerve damage in the feet and lower limbs, result in the majority of the over 40,000 toe, foot, and leg amputations annually in the United States, and four of our interviewees have already lost one or more toes or a foot. Only one interviewee mentioned having problems with erectile dysfunction (although it wasn't one of our usual questions to ask, so the incidence could be higher). In men who have yet to be diagnosed with diabetes, erectile dysfunction is often a symptom of diabetes and/or vascular problems.

You may or may not already know that diabetes can also accelerate the development of heart and other vascular diseases. The leading cause of death in all Americans is the same for people with diabetes: heart disease. If you have diabetes, though, your risk of dying from a heart attack is elevated. Many undiagnosed people with type 2 diabetes first learn of their condition shortly after having their first heart attack. At that point, they likely have already had diabetes for a number of years without knowing it, but long enough for it to cause significant damage. In their case, ignorance of diabetes is certainly not bliss, but an estimated one-third of all people with type 2 diabetes currently remain undiagnosed even though their elevated blood sugars are doing damage over time. Cardiovascular problems are very common in type 2 diabetes, but their incidence can be reduced significantly with more effective blood sugar control. For type 1s, intensive diabetes management has also been shown to reduce their risk of cardiovascular disease.

Plaque buildup in the coronary arteries begins in childhood, and when you have other commonly occurring health problems, like high blood pressure and elevated cholesterol levels to go along with diabetes, heart disease can progress more rapidly. Unfortunately, almost three-fourths of adults with diabetes have high blood pressure (with readings above 140 over 90 mm Hg) that may not be effectively controlled with medications, and most have abnormal levels of blood fats and cholesterol. Of the more than thirty-five people that we interviewed for this book who have had diabetes longer than 40 years, seven had already undergone coronary bypass surgery for blocked arteries, and another had had angioplasty in his leg vessels to improve blood flow to his feet. Strokes are also more commonplace in people with diabetes, although only three of our interviewees has been affected by a stroke: one was a minor one that impacted part of his vision in one eye (optic nerve damage); the second was resolved with a clot-busting drug, leaving no lasting problems; and the third one has affected her ability to walk somewhat, but she still didn't need a wheelchair or a walker despite her advanced age.

Diabetes can cause other health problems that have the ability to severely limit your quality of life, even though they may not be as life-threatening. They include lesser-well-known complications like periodontal disease, joint issues (trigger finger, frozen shoulder, carpal tunnel syndrome, and tendonitis), thyroid gland problems, fungal infections (in toes), hammer toes (deformity of the second, third, or fourth toes where they are bent at the middle joint, usually caused by muscular imbalances), high arches, dry skin on heels, droopy eyelids, and more frequent infections, such as bladder and breast (e.g., blocked milk duct in lactating diabetic women), and poor pregnancy outcomes. Five of our interviewees have experienced some degree of periodontal (gum) disease (or at least thought to mention it as a related complication of diabetes), although only one had lost any of her teeth because of it. Many of the old-timers with diabetes have had some problems with trigger fingers (permanently curled fingers that have to be repaired surgically—six cases), carpal tunnel syndrome (five surgeries), or frozen shoulders (five cases), although other types of tendon inflammations are more common in people with diabetes as well. Thyroid gland problems have been diagnosed in four of our interviewees, along with at least one case of permanently droopy eyelids. Others may have hammer toes and dry skin in their heels (resulting in cracks that four people mentioned), but then again, not everyone associates these symptoms with diabetes and may not have thought to bring them up when asked about complications. Finally, in poorly controlled diabetic mothers with either preexisting diabetes or gestational onset, infants can experience a greater incidence of mild to severe birth defects, but none of our interviewees has experienced this problem.

❧ 11 ❧

Respect the Power of Diabetes

Seeing other people with diabetes who really don't take care of themselves and who are getting diabetic complications can be a very motivating experience. If nothing else, it should teach you to respect the power of poorly controlled diabetes, which can easily ravage your body and steal your good health and longevity. You can also use your fear of diabetic complications to your advantage by letting it motivate you to maintain control over your blood glucose levels and to live a healthier life.

For many, fear of problems has been a major motivating factor throughout their diabetic lives. When Barbara Baxter, a resident of Yorktown, Virginia, who has been living with diabetes for 53 years, was first diagnosed at the age of 12, she remembers that her doctor told her, "If you don't take care of yourself, you won't live past 16." She has never forgotten this dire warning she was given, and she has kept it in the back of her mind all these years. For Karen Poenisch, her biggest fear is just that she will have a heart attack brought on by diabetes. "I try to do things proactively to prevent problems," she says, "but I still worry about it."

Don Gifford had a second cousin who died from diabetic complications at the age of 14, and he knew of others in his hometown with diabetes-related kidney problems. "I assumed growing up that I would have all sorts of complications and wouldn't grow very old. When I survived to be an adult, I worried if I was going to be around to pay my child's college tuition." (He was.) He also remembers visiting the Cleveland Clinic as a kid and sitting in the waiting room there with older, blind diabetic adults and others with leg stumps due to amputations. He has used his tremendous fear of complications to lead him to live a healthier life with diabetes, and to date, he has only suffered some problems with diabetic retinopathy correctable with laser treatments more than 15 years ago, despite a rebellious period from the age of 13 to 29 when he knows his control was much worse. "You have to figure out when it matters and when it doesn't," he says. He finds himself in a state of disbelief now when he sees people with diabetes who don't choose to take care of themselves. To him, diabetes control definitely matters.

Similarly, Bob Cleveland worried about getting complications. "In grammar and junior high school, my principal lost a leg due to diabetes. When I found that out, I wondered when it was going to happen to me." Although she has had diabetes less long than Bob, Mary Sue Rubin also remarks that the fear of complications can be a motivating factor. "When I was younger, I had no fear of diabetes, but I worry about it more now since I've had more diabetes education. Seeing other people with diabetes who really don't take care of themselves and have health problems because of it is very motivating." She believes that you should use your fear to help motivate yourself to live a healthier life.

Freddi Fredrickson, who was diagnosed with diabetes in her late teens and lives in Shadow Hills in Southern California, has worried about getting complications for most of her 46 years with diabetes. "I was sure I would have kidney failure," she recalls, "which caused me lots of fear and trepidation. After about the first 15 years with diabetes, I had one urine test that was a little off. The doctor told me, 'Maybe you have kidney disease,' but what I heard was, 'You have kidney disease.' It was like a 'come to Jesus' moment for me. I became diligent about my diabetes care then, taking four shots a day, and my kidney parameters are still normal."

In Larry Verity's early search for information back in the 1970s when he was diagnosed, the available knowledge was that diabetes was going to reduce your life expectancy by a third. He started out fearful of losing his vision and his ability to function and worried about needing to go on kidney dialysis. He used this fear, though, to motivate him to try to limit his possibility of developing them, and so far he is complication-free after more than 31 years with diabetes. So is Chuck Eichten after a similar number of years with diabetes. Chuck says that when he was first diagnosed as a teenager, the nurses at the hospital who were helping with his education put the fear of God in him by telling him about all the things that can go wrong with you—like amputated legs. "I took it as a personal challenge," Chuck recalls. "I didn't stress about it every minute of the day, but it was a driving factor in the care I still take of myself."

Ron DeNunzio, however, had to find out about the power of complications in a much harder way: He had to have a part of both of his feet and lower limbs amputated after he had only had diabetes for about 20 years. He says, "I look back on my life as a learning experience with lots of messing up. I think I fell twenty-two times and got up twenty-four times. My complications have made me a stronger person, a better person."

Not everyone has worried extensively about getting complications, though. Patty Schaeffer's only fear was for her vision because she's admittedly a bookworm. "Other than that, I had no fear. If they were going to happen, they were going to happen," she says.

Carolyn Balcom is also aware of the possibility of complications, and she has seen some people with severe ones, but her approach is to do the best she can to take care of herself. "I'm not going to spend all my time worrying about them," she states, "but you do have to respect diabetes and how much damage it can cause." So far, after living with diabetes for 43 years, the only complication she has experienced is some mild gastroparesis. "I'm not expecting bad things, but you have to know this possibility exists."

Similarly, Judy Tripathi is a "robust diabetic" with no real complications even after 43 years of diabetes herself. She admits that she used to think about complications more when she worked for 16 years in a dialysis clinic (where many of the patients had diabetes) than she does now. "I don't think about complications now," she says. "I guess I'm not preoccupied with it because I know I'm doing the best that I can." She does admit, though, that she uses her diabetes to keep her perspective, inspiration, and desire to maintain her health and longevity.

❦ 12 ❧

Control Your Problems before They Control You

I t is entirely possible for you to learn how to prevent and control diabetic health problems before they happen to you. A quote from John Rodosevich, a resident of San Diego, California, who has been living with diabetes for 42 of his 60 years, sums it all up: "There is no instant gratification in diabetes care. You just have to develop good habits early on to prevent complications." Nevertheless, both prevention and control of any problems that do arise involves finding out about the latest treatment and technologies available. For example, controlling the progression of kidney disease involves the use of ACE (angiotensin-converting enzyme) inhibitors, blood pressure medications, and better methods to keep your blood sugars in an optimal range. With such aggressive treatments, end-stage kidney problems, including dialysis and kidney transplants, are avoidable for many individuals, and kidney problems that are diagnosed early can often be kept at bay.

Either ACE inhibitors or another class of drugs known as ARBs (angiotensin receptor blockers) can slow early kidney disease by 30 to 70 percent. It's recommended that you have both your albumin levels in your urine and your blood creatinine levels measured annually to determine the degree of damage and the best course to follow. Although high-protein diets are not likely to cause kidney problems, consuming a protein-limited diet if you develop significant kidney damage is likely prudent.

Dr. Steve himself has been living well despite having significant protein found in his urine during laboratory testing done for a health insurance application back in 1989, but he takes both ACE inhibitors and blood pressure medications to protect his kidneys. Marc Blatstein has also been taking ACE inhibitors since the mid-1980s when he was diagnosed with kidney damage. To this day, his kidney function is in a great range, and his doctor is amazed at his current test results over 20 years after his initial diagnosis. (He also attributes some of his success in this regard to doing chelation therapy for the past 14 years, but such therapies have not been scientifically proven to be effective.) Freddi Fredrickson also religiously takes an ACE inhibitor to protect her kidney function, although her lab tests have remained normal for the past 30 years since her one abnormal result.

As an aside, you should know that it's possible to make your kidney function results (i.e., urinary microalbumin and protein, plasma creatinine, and creatinine clearance) appear abnormal with exercise. It is well documented, even in nondiabetic athletes, that a bout of moderate to heavy exercise can increase the output of protein in the urine through a process called "exercise-induced proteinuria." The best advice is to refrain from all exercise (other than your usual activities of daily living) when you are collecting a twenty-four-hour urine sample or going to the lab for a single sample urine test. By way of example, on one occasion almost 20 years ago and before Dr. Sheri knew about this phenomenon, she exercised moderately for an hour on the day she was collecting her urine, and her urinary protein levels came back abnormally high. To be certain about the diagnosis (which petrified her), she repeated the testing the next week without doing any exercise, and all of her kidney parameters were perfectly normal. Although she has also used her fear of kidney complications to her advantage since that time, a "false positive" test result is never enjoyable and is best prevented whenever possible.

Dr. Richard "Dick" Bernstein, a 73-year-old, 60-year veteran of diabetes who runs a booming diabetes practice in Mamaroneck, New York, knows from first-hand experience that many diabetic complications are actually reversible. "When I was diagnosed with diabetes back in 1946, I was put on a high-carb diet and it nearly killed me." He put himself on a low-carbohydrate version once he started getting significant complications in his 30s (after about 20 years with poorly controlled diabetes), but he reversed nearly all of the significant ones after several years of maintaining optimal blood glucose control. "Nerve problems get better, but musculoskeletal ones don't," he claims. "I still have some muscle wasting on the top of my feet, droopy eyelids, hammer toes, and high arches. Trigger point massage for one frozen shoulder helped years ago, but 20 years later when the other one got it, it was too late—it was not reversed. The severe proteinuria that I had developed on the high-carb diet is long gone, though, as are my cardiomyopathy and my elevated blood lipid levels." He shared that with excellent blood sugar control, he was also able to reverse the calcification of the muscle layer in the walls of his arteries that had been prematurely aging his blood vessels, a complication that can lead to heart disease. "Optimally, you should have no spikes in your blood sugar—meaning that your glucose levels should be normal at all times like other people. That's the way to be a survivor."

Certain complications like gastroparesis, a slowing of stomach emptying after a meal caused by central nerve damage, can make it harder to control blood sugars after eating. A slower than expected rate of carbohydrate absorption can cause people with it to get low blood sugar after eating and taking insulin, only to wind up with too high of levels later on. "I try to only eat moderate amounts of carbs," says Patricia La France-Wolf, who suffers from this problem. "I can't limit my carbs too extremely, though, with gastroparesis. I limit myself to about eighty grams or less a day, or about thirty per meal, because I have noticed that if I eat more, I have a hard time keeping my sugars down, even when I bolus frequently with my insulin pump." Dr. Steve, who also suffers from mild gastroparesis, finds that using Symlin to additionally slow down the rate at which his stomach empties after a meal also helps him, although its use is usually not recommended for people with this condition. (Read about Symlin and how it works in more detail in Secret 31.) To control her symptoms, Vena Petrotta uses Reglan, a prescription medication that she feels has been very beneficial. Both are available only by prescription, though, so you would need to talk with your physician about the possibility of using either to treat this problem.

Other nerve problems, specifically peripheral ones rather than central, can cause pain or numbness in your feet and legs and occasionally arms and hands, which may be controllable with certain medications like Cymbalta, Neurontin, and Lyrica (also available by prescription only). Interestingly, recent studies of diabetic people doing long-term aerobic exercise training found that it may prevent the onset or slow the progression of peripheral nerve damage, so exercising by itself may be a good preventative medicine for many of these potential complications.

To care for your eyes and detect changes early when problems are more easily treated, have a dilated eye exam performed annually, ideally by an ophthalmologist. Most people with diabetes go blind because they are seen by an eye doctor too late, since most cases are preventable. The general rule of thumb is that if you develop diabetes in childhood, you should have your eyes checked by the time you reach puberty (around age 13). Everyone else should have an eye exam right after being diagnosed with diabetes.

Undoubtedly, some eye problems are easier to treat than others. For Grant McArthur, his diabetes diagnosis at the age of 21 back in 1965 involved a reversible loss of his sight. He had gone into the Army and was in training in Ft. Lewis, Washington, to be sent over to Vietnam, when he started to have extreme pain in the back of his eyes for several days. Then he lost his sight completely. At the hospital when they tested his blood sugar for the first time, it was off the charts. After six to seven months in the Army hospital and a course of steroid treatment for his eyes, his sight came back. However, when your sight is reduced from hemorrhages inside your eyes caused by the growth of unstable new vessels (proliferative diabetic retinopathy), the treatment usually consists of laser burns to the peripheral parts of the back of the eye (retina), along with a vitrectomy to surgically remove the cloudy vitreous fluid in your eyes if they fail to clear out on their own. In the case of Rich Humphreys, a vitrectomy restored one eye's vision that he had been without for a year and a half. In other cases, as with Natalie Saunders, retinopathy has proliferated and only caused vision loss in one eye (at least initially). After having laser surgery and a vitrectomy in her left eye, she had some laser surgery done on her right (unaffected) eye as well. "We were just putting it in the bank," she says.

Certain other problems like cardiovascular ones can be controlled through early intervention, dietary and exercise interventions, medications to control blood pressure and cholesterol levels, angioplasty, placement of arterial stents (to open up coronary arteries), bypass surgery, and more. Aspirin therapy is also recommended for most adults with diabetes, along with smoking cessation. In the case of any vascular problems, early intervention —before you have a heart attack or stroke—can greatly lower your chances of dying early or having debilitating health problems, so get checked out regularly, particularly if you start to experience any symptoms of reduced blood flow to any part of your body. Chest pain at rest or during exertion, shortness of breath, and pain in your legs with walking are all potential signs of cardiovascular problems that should be checked out as soon as possible.

Also, if you're experiencing a stroke and can get to a hospital within a three-hour window from the onset of symptoms to receive a clot-busting drug called tPA (tissue plasminogen activator), your outcome can be much more favorable. Jim Arthur experienced a stroke, but was able to get a dose of tPA in time, and he has no lasting signs of ever having had reduced blood flow to his brain as a result. A sudden loss of vision, a sudden inability to walk or stand, or a sudden slurring of your words can be a symptom of a stroke, and you should be checked out immediately by a physician. Antiplatelet agents, such as aspirin and Plavix, and anticoagulants like Coumadin, interfere with the blood's ability to clot and can play an important role in preventing stroke. However, if you have stomach ulcers or already take other anti-inflammatory drugs like Advil, you should take no more than a baby aspirin (80 mg) a day, but for others, 325 mg of a coated aspirin like Ecotrin may be a more effective stroke preventative.

For annoying, but not potentially fatal, complications like frozen joints, trigger fingers, and other types of tendonitis, the best solutions vary. Frozen shoulder (known medically as "adhesive capsulitis," caused by chronic inflammation or injury and resulting in a significant loss of range of motion of the shoulder in all directions) can often be treated with trigger point massage and physical therapy. Jessica Ching comments that although she went to more than 100 physical therapy sessions last year, she can still run, and she trains for half marathons eight months out of the year. For others, frozen joints (which includes shoulders primarily, but also hips) slow them down for a while, but they don't knock them out for good. Trigger fingers that result in excessive curling can be treated surgically, which many people with diabetes have had to undergo on more than one digit. For other joint or tendon inflammation, prophylactic use of anti-inflammatory medications like ibuprofen and aspirin may work to control pain and stiffness before they limit your activities.

Interestingly, some people with diabetes have also turned to herbal remedies and supplements to try to control their problems, particularly ones related to neuropathy. Although Anna Maria Gould says that omega-3 fatty acid supplements (found normally in oily fish, flaxseed, and certain nuts) help when she gets tendonitis, along with glucosamine supplements, Marc Blatstein uses omega-3s to counteract the effects of peripheral neuropathy. Rich Humphreys, however, swears by quercetin, one of the natural phytonutrients from plants called flavonoids, to control the neuropathy (numbness in his case) that had been slowly developing in his legs. "I had neuropathy in one leg for eight years that was cured by quercetin," he claims. "Within three years of taking it, the neuropathy had gone to half, and then it was completely gone in another six months. I know the herb did it because when

I stopped taking it for a short while, my neuropathy came back." If you'd rather get more of this flavonoid naturally, quercetin-rich consumables include cocoa, red grapes and wine, apples (especially the peel), apricots, green beans, blueberries, blackberries, raspberries, bog whortleberries and all sorts of other less common berries, broccoli, buckwheat, celery, cherries, cranberries, fennel leaves, kale, lettuce (all types), onions, most hot peppers, plums, dill weed, spinach, sweet potato leaves, tarragon, black and green teas (especially brewed from leaves), tomatoes (particularly cherry) and tomato products, watercress, and bee pollen.

Along a similar vein, the use of alpha-lipoic acid, a strong antioxidant compound found naturally in foods like spinach, may also reduce the symptoms of neuropathy in the feet and hands (e.g., burning, pain, and numbness) when taken as a supplement. Jim Arthur had been taking Cymbalta and Neurontin, both of which are used to treat painful neuropathy, but they also cause dizziness, a problem he has recently been experiencing. After a visit with a neuropathy specialist, Jim is now instead trying a recommended cocktail of antioxidants, including alpha-lipoic acid, borage oil (high in gamma linolenic acid, also found in evening primrose oil), benfotiamine (a derivative of thiamine, or vitamin B1), and vitamin C. Antioxidants are believed to be integrally involved in the prevention of many diabetic complications, such as cataracts, which result at least partially from deficient glutathione levels leading to a faulty antioxidant defense system within the lens of your eye. Nutrients such as alpha-lipoic acid, vitamins E and C, and selenium can increase your levels of glutathione and its activity, allowing for better protection of your eyes and other tissues. Taking too much of these disease-fighting compounds in the form of large supplemental doses can be counterproductive, though, as almost all antioxidants have been shown to have the opposite effect when taken in unnaturally large doses, so it's best not to go overboard when taking them or any prescribed medications. It's also best to let your physician know about any herbal remedies you're using, since they can potentially interact with prescribed medications and cause bad side effects. The scientific findings about such herbal and vitamin remedies are not conclusive currently, so Dr. Steve is hesitant to officially "prescribe" any of these for his patients.

JAMES W. QUANDER, AGE 86 (DECEASED IN 2004), LIVING WITH TYPE 1 DIABETES FOR 80+ YEARS

If there ever was a diabetic trailblazer, the honor should go to James William Quander, a recently deceased, lifetime resident of Washington, D.C. What makes him unique—other than his long life with diabetes—is the fact that he was an African American, the longest-living one with type 1 diabetes on record. Born in 1918, he was diagnosed with diabetes shortly before reaching the age of 6 when a sickness "episode" put him in the hospital. At that time, his parents realized that he had gone through a similar illness at the age of 3, so he likely had actually had diabetes for longer than his 80 years on insulin that started early in 1924. At the time of his diagnosis, there were few specialists available to treat diabetes and even fewer with doctors' admitting privileges at Children's Hospital, the local pediatric hospital in the D.C. area. As a result, young James was usually the only juvenile patient at Freedman's Hospital (now called Howard University Hospital), the local adult hospital founded in 1863 to take care of the freed slaves and their descendants, and the only one where his doctor, also African American, could care for him due to segregation laws in place at the time.

By all medical accounts, young James was supposed to be dead by the age of 10, or at least his parents received that message from his doctors. They chose not to pass on their expectation of an early demise to their son, telling him instead that he had a very serious illness that he would have to work hard to manage and they were doing all they could to give him the same quality of life his four siblings had. Given the racial segregation of Washington, D.C., from the time of his diagnosis through the 1940s (and beyond), he had to deal repeatedly with double discrimination. His race kept him from gaining better, higher-paying jobs, and his diabetes was viewed as a potentially contagious disease that led many of his peers to shun him. He could not join an ROTC program because the bayonet rifles used were "dirty" and could possibly cut him and cause an infection that would not heal due to diabetes. He applied for a position with the FBI, but he was told at the time that he only qualified to work for the postal service because of his skin color. Despite starting out at a lowly postal worker job, he ultimately worked for the U.S. Federal Government for 33 years as an economist, statistician, computer programmer, and manpower labor specialist.

For the most part, James chose to keep his diabetes a secret, not publicly coming out of the "diabetes closet" until the 1970s when he was already in his fifties. Diabetes awareness at that time had finally reached a point where most people realized it was not a communicable condition. Of special note, he was ordained as one of the first of sixteen Permanent Deacons in the Roman Catholic Church in 1971 when the Permanent Diaconate was revived after an eight-hundred-year hiatus. Then, in September of 1975 on a trip to Rome, he served as sole assistant to Pope Paul VI in celebrating a daily mass. Throughout his later years, he was also active in tracing the history of the Quander family, one of the oldest African American families in the United States with lineage dating back to 1684. Originating in Ghana, a branch of his family had been slaves owned by George Washington (freed by Martha as decreed in the president's will), while others had been freed shortly after their arrival in America.

James was married to his wife, Joherra Rohulamin Quander, for three days short of 60 years (when she died unexpectedly). In another trailblazing moment, James had married her despite the fact that 1940s society was almost completely segregated, and her family came from East Asian/European roots, not African American. He told everyone, "I didn't pick my family, but I plan to pick my wife." She bore him four healthy children, three boys and one girl, none who has diabetes (his ten grandchildren and two great-grandchildren are also diabetes-free).

A fervent believer that anyone can manage his or her diabetes, James had five simple words that he lived by: faith, hope, love, perseverance, and discipline. For him, "faith" constituted his own faith in God and in himself. As for "hope," he always maintained the hope that diabetes would be cured in his lifetime. In his later years when it was apparent that a cure was unlikely for him, he put his energy into using available management tools to control his blood sugars and teaching others to do the same. "Love" meant that love given to and received from his family and friends over his lifetime also sustained him, particularly when his disease was troublesome. He felt "perseverance" gave him the determination to live life to the fullest in spite of having diabetes, and he passed this character trait on to his children. Finally, "discipline" topped the list as the most important word, and he was undeniably disciplined in caring for his disease for over eight decades.

His oldest son, Judge Rohulamin Quander, set out to help his father document the unique details of his remarkable life, culminating in a 2006 coauthored book called *The Quander Quality: The True Story of a Black Trailblazing Diabetic* (www.TheQuanderQuality.com). James insisted that when publicizing the book after his death, his son donate half of all proceeds to Howard University College of Medicine for diabetes education and research. In so many ways, his is a story that will continue to inspire people for many years to come.

PART THREE

Control Secrets

Know Your Numbers and Assume Nothing

O ne characteristic of all the longest-living people with diabetes is that they all started using blood glucose meters religiously not long after they became widely available in the early 1980s. The key is really not only to know your numbers (which you should never assume that you know without testing), but also to know what to do with them, which is a large part of the knowledge acquisition advocated by Dr. Steve's TCOYD organization. You can use frequent testing to detect patterns and to learn your body's unique response to different things—foods, activities, medications, emotional and physical stress, and more—so that you can adjust your medications or insulin to work for you as effectively as possible to control your blood glucose and prevent future complications.

The present and future of glucose monitoring are far brighter than the pre-meter past. "Before meters, all monitoring methods still made you guess what your sugars actually were. Now, in five seconds time, you can know. There have been great advances in diabetes in the past 80 years," says Bob Cleveland. A lot of people have also learned that their guesses were way off before, although they assumed they knew what their blood glucose was. "When I used to get high blood glucose levels a lot, when I was near normal, they felt low," remarks Patricia La France-Wolf. Similarly, Carolyn Balcom admits, "When I thought I was low, I might be right or might not be. I had a tendency to overeat whenever I felt low. Blood glucose meters showed that I didn't need much to bring my sugars up." Vena Petrotta comments, "I got the first meter when it was available. Urine testing was no way to test blood sugars. Whenever I felt sick (whether I was high or low), they used to give me Coke." John Rodosevich agrees. "In the early years I had diabetes, my trips to the doctor were frustrating. I'd get blood work done and find out my results six months later. Until we all started monitoring our blood glucose, we didn't make much progress in diabetes care."

In reality, it's not always easy to tell right away if your blood glucose level is too high or too low right when you start feeling "funny." In fact, when your blood sugar is changing rapidly—either going up or down—you often can't tell which way it's going until your symptoms progress. Moreover, if you've been running high for a while and your blood sugar starts to decrease rapidly, you can feel hypoglycemic even when your blood sugar is still elevated. As Larry Verity wisely advises, "Never assume that you're low—you may actually be hyperglycemic. Always check your blood sugar first before you treat it."

Freddi Fredrickson additionally recommends doing a lot of blood glucose testing to stay in control. "Seeing what your blood sugar is can be a good incentive to stay in control and feel better," she says. "I just really worry about the lows, and I'm constantly vigilant for hypoglycemia. Testing helps you figure out what your carb ratio is and how much one unit of insulin lowers you." Since

Jim Turner also experiences lows that he doesn't always feel, he checks his blood sugars at least twelve times a day. "You can only treat it when you know what it is," he says, adding, "and we're so lucky we can test it. I don't mind it at all. I look at it as a gift, a way to find out something that I don't necessarily know." Natalie Saunders checks hers whenever she feels she needs to know or wants to verify her blood glucose. "Sometimes I feel low, and I'll be 154 or 94." There's sometimes no way to know for certain which one you are without testing. Gladys Dull checks hers at least three times a day, more if she's not feeling right, although she doesn't adjust her insulin levels often because her diet is very consistent.

WHAT SHOULD YOUR NUMBERS BE? HERE ARE THE RECOMMENDED TARGET GOALS FOR BLOOD GLUCOSE, GLYCATED HEMOGLOBIN, CHOLESTEROL, AND BLOOD PRESSURE

	Fasting (Overnight)	Other Times
Blood glucose (mg/dl)	70—120 (before all meals)	<180 (2 hours after meals)
Glycated hemoglobin (HbA1c) (%)	<7.0 (American Diabetes Association goal)	<6.5 (American Association of Clinical Endocrinologists)
Total cholesterol (mg/dl)	<200	<180 (even better)
HDL-cholesterol (mg/dl)	>40 for males, >50 for females	>60 (optimal for everyone)
LDL-cholesterol (mg/dl)	<100 (for diabetes)	<70 (for higher heart disease risk)
Triglycerides (mg/dl)	<150	
Blood pressure (mm Hg)	<120/<80	Never over 130/85

As for other health-related numbers, Dee Brehm advises monitoring your blood pressure and cholesterol levels carefully as well. Bernadette McIntyre agrees. "You need to keep up with all of your medical stuff," she advises, "including seeing your podiatrist (foot doctor), diabetes doctor, and dentist to have your teeth cleaned and checked. Take advantage of good medical help to control all aspects of your health." Admittedly, it's a lot to keep track of. As Natalie Saunders says, "It's not easy watching my carbs, triglycerides, and cholesterol."

Other than managing blood glucose levels, cholesterol gets the most attention. Many people are already taking cholesterol-lowering medications, the most popular of which are "statins," such as Lipitor, Crestor, and Zocor. Not only do statins lower the "bad" LDL-cholesterol, but they also appear to help protect cardiovascular health by preventing blood clots from forming (a common precipitator of heart attack and stroke), improve blood flow (endothelial function), and lower systemic inflammation. Although these medications save lives, they aren't the only way to lower blood cholesterol levels. Getting more exercise, improving your diet, controlling your blood sugars, and getting plenty of fiber all help reduce cholesterol, often just as effectively as taking additional medications without the cost or the side effects. Regardless of how you achieve it, the goal of all of these measurements is, of course, to maintain your health in an optimal range throughout your life. So, strive to maintain your blood glucose levels (and blood fats and pressure) in a normal range (or as near to normal as you can get) at all times, but keep your control in perspective and don't let it become obsessive or life-altering in a bad way, which can have the opposite effect on your health. It's a fine balancing act, but the future is still bright with upcoming improvements in care and measuring tools and devices.

🌿 14 🌿

Vary Your Glucose Testing

Whether you have type 1 diabetes or type 2, testing your blood sugars at different times, more inconsistently than just before meals and at bedtime, can often reveal trends with your blood glucose levels that might not be apparent otherwise. Since studies now indicate the post-meal glucose excursions may be as important in causing diabetic complications as overall glucose control, controlling such spikes may be the key to preventing microvascular complications like diabetic retinopathy. Thus, testing not just before meals but occasionally one hour and two hours afterward can let you know how your various meals are affecting your blood glucose levels and how much variability in your glucose levels you are usually experiencing. Both the American Diabetes Association and the American Association of Clinical Endocrinologists recommend checking two hours after your first bite of a meal. They haven't changed that recommendation yet, but we now know that people with either type of diabetes reach a peak seventy-two minutes after eating with a variation of twenty-three minutes either way—based on the results of continuous glucose monitoring.

The best idea, then, is to vary your blood glucose testing instead of just testing before meals and at bedtime. "If you don't know what your blood sugars are," Barbara Baxter asks, "how can you know how much insulin to give?" Frankly, you can't. "You name it—I test it," says Carol Sawyer, a 61-year-old resident of Portsmouth, Virginia, who has been living with diabetes for 49 years. "If it doesn't feel right, I test it." She also tests before every meal and at bedtime as well. Peter Gariti tests at least four times a day also, but says that if he's high before a meal, he tests again afterward. Likewise, since hypoglycemia is such a big concern for Carol Sessions, she checks her blood sugars a lot and tries to learn her body's response to different types of foods. "I avoid eating things that make my sugar shoot up," she says. To find out which foods do, she has to test both before and varied times after eating on many occasions.

"If I eat a lot of carbs or something new," says Freddi Fredrickson, "I do extra glucose testing for two to four hours afterwards. Testing so much really helps to find trends." In a similar manner, Bernadette McIntyre checks very frequently, usually ten to twelve times a day including after meals, and gives extra insulin (one to two units) to cover any elevations in her blood glucose. "I always try to cover everything I eat," she says. "Even if it means I have to check my sugar after eating, I never let it go too high."

Bob Elder agrees that testing at differing times of the day is a key to being in control. "I'm very aggressive as far as keeping my blood glucose below 150," he states. "I hate it when it gets high—I dwell on that more than the lows. That's why I check my blood sugar at least five or more times a day. If I have any question or I'm on the road, I will check it then, too." When Dr. Sheri got her first blood glucose meter in the mid-1980s, she used to check all the time—sometimes even hourly during the whole day—just to learn the glycemic effects of different foods and activities. In attempting to be in optimal control both before and during all her pregnancies, she often checked her blood sugars both before and one and two hours after eating, sometimes even more often. "Testing frequently and at different times is the only way to really learn how your body responds and to optimize your control," she says. "I know myself very well because of all the testing I have done." She tests even more often when she's doing something outside of her normal routines, such as traveling or trying out a new physical activity. Dr. Steve's advice to people is also to "test, test, test," and "know what to do with the numbers," and his fellow Southern Californian Larry Verity agrees that the more you check your blood glucose, the more you know.

Some people check more often for reasons of safety, such as to catch low blood sugars before they can become a problem. Since Grant McArthur's bad car accident due to hypoglycemia, he has been checking more frequently anytime he is traveling. "I check my blood sugar every time before I head out the door," he says, "and again while I'm out." Jane Dohrmann also says, "I test at least five times a day and as many as twelve to fifteen, depending on what's going on with me and my blood sugars." Similarly, Matt Besley tests eight to fourteen times a day, particularly to stay in control when he's doing a lot of surfing. He says, "You have to monitor frequently but inconsistently to know what's going on with your body." He also runs his blood sugars in a tight range and gets low "way more often than the average person with diabetes." He admits that he needs to find a way to avoid having lows so often because he has a young daughter that he's often responsible for looking after.

Living with type 2 diabetes, Zach Barneis is less likely to experience lows than some other people, but he still tests in the morning, before each meal, and whenever he feels a little hypoglycemic or if he feels too high, demonstrating that even type 2s on insulin can benefit from additional and varied testing. If you don't use insulin, it's still important to see what effect different foods and activities are having on your blood sugars, though. You can have fairly good overall control, but still be experiencing post-meal spikes that could cause problems over time and be more effectively controlled with another medication that you might not yet be using.

❧ 15 ❧

Learn How to Prevent Bad Lows

Hypoglycemia (usually defined as a blood glucose level below 65 mg/dl) is an unavoidable consequence of tight blood glucose control and is much more common in insulin users than people controlled with oral medications alone. Certain situations can increase the likelihood of experiencing low blood sugars, including drinking more than a couple of alcoholic drinks in the previous twelve hours, emotional stress or depression, a hypoglycemic episode in the past twenty-four to forty-eight hours, recent vigorous or prolonged exercise, a rapid drop in blood sugars (for any reason), and reduced food intake. Most people who have had diabetes for longer than 10 years have a blunted release of glucose-raising hormones (e.g., glucagon and adrenaline) in response to insulin-induced hypoglycemia. Experiencing bad low blood sugar reactions is one of the main factors lowering diabetic individuals' quality of life. Even the fear of such lows is enough to make your anxiety levels higher. As Anna Maria Gould states succinctly for all type 1s and type 2s on insulin, "Lows are a big problem."

Mild hypoglycemic reactions are not pleasurable, but at least they're easy to treat with carbohydrate intake, but if your blood sugars drop too low without symptoms or enough time to react and treat it, you may become unresponsive or unconscious. If you ever get bad lows without being aware of it, you may have a condition known as "hypoglycemia unawareness," which may affect up to about 20 percent or more of insulin users. Although it's less common in people with type 2 diabetes, if they are experiencing it, unawareness is associated with a higher incidence of severe episodes of hypoglycemia.

Normally, when your blood sugars start to get too low, you will experience symptoms—such as sweating, shaking, weakness, visual changes, and others—that are caused by the release of adrenaline and the other glucose-raising hormones. If you're unaware, though, you may have either milder or missing symptoms due to a blunted hormone release. Since low blood sugars affect your brain's cognitive abilities, you may even test your blood sugars when you're low and not realize that you need to eat, resist others' help when they try to give you something to treat it, or even run away from the paramedics trying to assist you. Hypoglycemia unawareness can occur at night (since people apparently wake up for less than half of their nighttime lows), but also during the day. Unless someone else is around to help recognize that you're very low and prompt you to treat it, serious problems like grand mal seizures and unconsciousness can result, neither of which is desirable in any way. As Chuck Eichten advises, "Don't have seizures." (Fortunately, he got rid of his by getting into tighter control on an insulin pump.)

Most people don't feel nearly as bad when their blood sugars are a little (or even a lot) high compared to when they're experiencing hypoglycemia; the greater unpleasantness of being low makes most people much more wary of them than highs. Even Gladys Dull admits that she lets her blood sugars run higher at night to prevent nighttime lows. "I only had bad lows when I was taking more insulin," she says, further commenting that she cut back on her insulin doses when the lows were frequent. Don Gifford ran himself high for many years (before getting a glucose meter) because of being afraid of running low and convulsing. Nevertheless, it's always better for your long-term health to try to keep your blood sugars normal and try to prevent lows rather than running blood sugars high to do so.

"I've only had three bad lows in 39 years of diabetes," says Will Speer, Sr., "but they always scared the living daylights out of me." By testing constantly (five to ten times daily), he finds that he doesn't get that low. For Bernadette McIntyre, checking her blood sugars frequently also allows her to pick up her lows before they get too bad, when she still is able to treat them and adjust the basal rate on her insulin pump down. Jane Dohrmann says that problems with bad lows have only been occurring for her over the past few years, even though she has had diabetes for over 40 years now, likely due to having a significant amount of insulin antibodies that make her blood sugars unpredictable at times. Vena Petrotta has been strict on her diet almost all of her years with diabetes for fear of complications, both longer-term ones and especially acute ones related to low blood glucose levels. "I always tried to stay on my diet," she says. "I was afraid of passing out like a friend of mine who had diabetes if I didn't."

Many people have experienced lows that are bad enough that they wake up either with paramedics standing over them or in the emergency room, such as the time when Grant McArthur's roommate had found him unconscious on the floor with his blood glucose level so low that it couldn't be measured. "It's scary at times," he admits, "but I have learned to live with it." Luckily for Bob Cleveland, he has experienced only one really scary incident with hypoglycemia in his 82 years with diabetes. "We used to spend summers camping out in national parks. On one trip out in the Rocky Mountains when we did lots of hiking up to the tundra where no trees were growing, my blood sugar got so low at the end of the day that I went into a coma." His companions had to call an ambulance into the park to treat him. "That one time made me realize that you really have to take special care with diabetes."

Other individuals have put their lives in jeopardy during bad hypoglycemic episodes. Carolyn Balcom only had one such low that resulted in her having a car accident. Barbara Baxter was also driving a car when she was very low and wound up in Hampton, Virginia (miles from her home), but she doesn't remember driving there. Luckily for her, someone driving nearby noticed that she was not doing well and got her to pull over in a church parking lot, where they called for an ambulance. The only thing she remembers about that incident is getting into her car. Similarly, Jim Arthur was pulled over by a police officer for weaving down the road in the car he was driving, but he doesn't even remember getting into it or driving anywhere. One time when Marialice Kern was driving, she lost consciousness due to an undetected low blood sugar, and she only came to after rear-ending another car on the interstate. Fortunately, no one was seriously hurt in that incident, but since that accident, she has had a rule to never take more than four units of rapid-acting insulin at any one time. Even Bill King experienced a minor traffic accident due to a hypoglycemic event.

THE LOWDOWN ON HYPOGLYCEMIA, DRIVING, AND YOUR RIGHT TO A DRIVER'S LICENSE

Losing consciousness due to a low blood glucose reaction while driving is certainly a major concern when it comes to staying alive and well, but it also becomes a legal issue when applying or reapplying for your driver's license. If you have had a bad hypoglycemic reaction that caused you to lose consciousness (even if you weren't driving at the time), you may have your license suspended for a period of time, depending on the regulations in your state. If your doctor does not know about your blackout from hypoglycemia and you weren't hospitalized from it, are you still obliged to admit to it if doing so may keep you from getting or renewing your driver's license? Legally, you have to check the "yes" box when asked, or you will be breaking the law by committing perjury on an official state document.

In Virginia where Dr. Sheri lives, the driver's license application specifically asks you whether (1) you have any physical or mental condition that requires medication, and (2) you have ever had a seizure, blackout, or loss of consciousness. If you answer "yes" to either of these two questions when applying for a driver's license, you must have a medical exam within the previous ninety days and an evaluation form filled out by your physician prior to receiving your license. Your doctor must state if you have experienced a recent blackout, but Virginia's Department of Motor Vehicles (DMV) also accept reports of potentially unsafe drivers from police officers, the courts, physicians, family members, friends, other citizens, and hospitals. At least in Virginia, there are no specific medical guidelines related to diabetes for noncommercial licenses except with regard to episodes of loss of consciousness for which they require that "drivers must be free of episodes for at least six months in order to be licensed."

Each state sets its own driving regulations, though. Some states apply strict rules to all drivers with diabetes, while many others apply them only to those who have actually experienced episodes of altered consciousness due to diabetes or its complications. Special licensing rules can include requirements for periodic medical evaluations from a physician and prohibitions on driving for a period of time after an episode of lost consciousness. The American Diabetes Association legal and advocacy department has compiled state-by-state regulations, which can be found on their Web site at www.diabetes.org/advocacy-and-legalresources/discrimination/drivers/pvt-driverslicenses.jsp. It's wise to learn what the specific laws are in your state.

As an alternate example, Dr. Steve's home state of California evaluates all cases individually and considers whether any loss of consciousness was an isolated episode or a chronic impairment. An isolated episode whose cause is related to conditions that are unlikely to recur (such as adverse reactions to medications) will typically not cause you to lose your license. However, if the episodes are part of a chronic or recurring condition (like hypoglycemic unawareness), they look at your degree of diabetes control afterward and the probability that you'll be able to maintain control of your blood sugars in the future. Generally, if you've been episode-free for three to six months, you can get a probationary license that requires regular monitoring by your physician and submission of follow-up medical reports to the DMV.

At least for some, improvements in certain driving rules have recently been implemented. A new transportation bill passed by Congress in 2005 required the U.S. Department of Transportation to amend its blanket ban against diabetic insulin users driving commercial vehicles (like trucks) in interstate commerce; the current rules allow for exemptions to this ban on a case-by-case basis. For example, exemptions have been given to drivers who have had no hypoglycemic reactions that resulted in loss of consciousness or seizure, that required the assistance of another person, or that resulted in impaired cognitive function without warning symptoms in the past five years (with one year of stability following any such episode). In each case, an endocrinologist has had to verify that the driver has demonstrated willingness to properly monitor and manage his or her diabetes, received education related to diabetes management, and is on a stable insulin regimen. In any case, though, put your and others' safety first and monitor your blood glucose levels closely whenever you're driving a car or commercial vehicle to prevent problems before they happen.

A worse scenario occurred when Grant McArthur hit a telephone pole when he went unconscious from a low while driving himself home one time. He broke his neck (but luckily not his spinal cord) and got whiplash from hitting it so hard. Other people have not been so lucky to have recoverable injuries or only one such life-threatening experience that caused them to lose consciousness. Dr. Sheri knew a diabetic teenager, the son of her mother's boss at the time, who drove his car into a tree and died as the result of a severe hypoglycemic reaction. Dick Bernstein also admits that he has had several car accidents as a result of bad hypoglycemia, but none of them caused him (or anyone else) serious injuries.

In addition, Dr. Steve, in his years of running TCOYD and being an endocrinologist, has also seen how devastating the effects of low blood sugars can be. Not long ago, he lost a good friend, patient, and TCOYD supporter, Cyndee Fena, who died from a severe, undetected hypoglycemic reaction that caused a fatal heart arrhythmia at night. He himself worries about the possibility of having an undetected nighttime low when he's traveling (which he does frequently) and staying alone in a hotel room. If you live alone or frequently travel by yourself, you may also be worried about experiencing undetected bad lows, with good reason. The best advice for anyone in a similar situation is to work diligently to prevent hypoglycemia (see tips in the "Low *Again?*" box), both during the day and at night. You may also want to consider running your blood glucose levels slightly higher at night if they usually go undetected. Some parents of type 1 diabetic children actually get up and test their kids' blood glucose levels during the night, and other single individuals have a friend or relative who calls them at a predetermined time daily to make sure they are cognitive enough to answer the phone. Alternately, using one of the new continuous glucose monitors that sound an alarm when your blood sugar goes low (see more on these monitors in Secret 35) may be a lifesaving decision.

Fortunately, you may actually be able to reverse hypoglycemia unawareness. Although it's common to experience diminished glucagon release when you get low if you've had diabetes for at least 2 to 10 years (a lesser release of which contributes to the condition), the most common reason why unawareness develops is having frequent low blood sugar reactions. One study found that after people slept through a low during the night (from which they eventually recovered without treatment), they were less likely to recognize a hypoglycemic episode the following day. Studies have also found, however, that normal hypoglycemic symptoms can be restored if you avoid all lows for a three-week period. So, if you do have a low reaction, try to avoid having another one for at least two days to retain a better awareness of your next one. In addition, some educators offer hypoglycemia unawareness training, which can teach you to become more aware of changes in your blood glucose levels. For many individuals with this problem, continuous glucose-monitoring devices may also help you recognize downward trends or rapid decreases in your blood glucose levels before they get to a critical point.

Although not routinely done nowadays, some individuals were forced by their doctors to experience their first hypoglycemic reaction under medical supervision—to learn what they feel like. Grant McArthur was still in the Army hospital when they brought his blood sugar down low enough for him to get symptoms so that he would know what if felt like. "I knew what to look for after that," he says. Early on, Jim Turner's doctor also made him experience a low blood glucose reaction by holding his lunch past the usual eating time. "My doctor wanted my first one to be in a hospital," he recalls. "He always tried to foster my independence. I was 17 when I got diabetes, and he made my parents butt out so that I could learn how to handle it myself." For him, though, the threat of daily lows is his biggest diabetes complication, as they often come on hard and fast, and he doesn't always get symptoms until he's very low. Bill King has similar problems with not always sensing his lows, particularly after long workouts.

LOW *AGAIN*? KEYS TO PREVENTING HYPOGLYCEMIA

- Know yourself—your body's reaction to specific foods, activities, and stress—by frequently monitoring your blood sugars until you learn your unique patterns and trends.
- Test your blood sugars more frequently whenever you're doing new activities, traveling, or are out of your usual routine.
- If you dose with rapid-acting insulin for food intake, learn how

much insulin you need for a certain intake of carbohydrate so that you don't overdose on insulin.

- Keep the "insulin on board" rules in mind, meaning that it takes at least two hours for most rapid-acting insulins to clear your bloodstream; if chasing a high with insulin, wait awhile for it to exert its full effects before taking more.

- Never skip meals or food for which you have already taken insulin or medications.

- If you're not sure when you'll eat (like in a restaurant), don't take all of your insulin before the food arrives; rather, wait until you have it in front of you.

- Follow your blood sugars for several hours after exercise to catch and prevent post-exercise delayed-onset hypoglycemia.

- Eat a carbohydrate snack (at least fifteen grams) within an hour after doing strenuous or prolonged exercise to help restore your muscles' glycogen more rapidly, along with a little protein and/or fat that will stick around longer.

Almost everyone who uses insulin has at least one "bad low" story, although sometimes they're more entertaining after the fact than worrisome. For example, Gladys Dull has a very protective dog, a Schipperke (pronounced "skipper key"), a breed known for "making an excellent and faithful watchdog." Her dog takes its role as her protector to a bit of an extreme, though. One time, when one of the women helping cook her meals had to call 911 to assist Gladys with a low blood sugar, the dog stood at the doorway and refused to let the paramedic come in to the house to treat her. Her neighbor was finally able to move the dog out of the way by force, but it took a bite out of his cheek in the process.

Also, take the bad low story of Jim Turner. In a dream one night, he believed that if he thought about going somewhere, he would simply go there and be there. When he woke up from this "think it, go there, be there" dream with low blood sugar, he thought the dream was real. His wife tried to give him some juice, but instead he jumped up on their bed, did a forward flip, and landed on it (somehow without injuring himself). His wife ran out of the room, and he chased her until he finally started to come out of it. (Maybe all the running increased his adrenaline levels, which would have raised his blood sugar.) Although it's not quite as funny as Jim's story, Dr. Sheri has seen someone attempt to program a clock radio with the TV remote when severely hypoglycemic. Overall, though, most low blood sugar episodes are not so entertaining to live through, and preventing them from occurring in the first place is one key to living long and well with diabetes.

❧ 16 ❧

Treat Your Lows Effectively (and with Good Taste)

Low blood sugar reactions can be treated with a number of foods and drinks, but the favorite appears to be glucose tablets. For those of you with diabetes less than about 15 years, you probably don't remember the original glucose tablets, which tasted just like chalk. Thankfully, they've come a long way since then. In addition to the more traditional orange variety, you can now get snazzy flavors, like watermelon, tropical fruit, coconut, sour apple, strawberry cream, grape, and raspberry.

Glucose tablets have a couple of benefits for treating lows that other substances don't have. For starters, glucose is the sugar that shows up in the bloodstream most rapidly, basically because it's what blood glucose is. By way of comparison, other sugars like fructose found in fruit have to be converted by your body into glucose and therefore have a slower effect. Another benefit is that glucose tablets come in precisely measured amounts—usually four grams of glucose per tablet—which makes it very easy to consume a specific number of grams of carbohydrates without overdoing it. With a little trial and error, you can easily determine how much each four-gram tablet is likely to raise your blood glucose level. "One glucose tablet raises mine 15 mg/dl," Dee Brehm states. "I do better using them so I don't overeat. The only time I feel really hungry is when I'm low." Marc Blatstein agrees. "When I was low, I used to eat everything in sight. Now, I just use glucose tablets or liquids with sugar, and I almost never over treat." Taking in too much to treat a low is an easy way to get yourself on a glucose "roller coaster," where you end up bouncing between being too low and ending up too high from the treatment. You can also use glucose gels (like InstaGlucose), but they typically contain higher amounts of carbohydrate.

According to our interviewees, other favorites to treat lows are juice (orange, apple, grape, pineapple, and cranberry), skim milk, sugared sodas, whole fruits (like bananas, apples, and grapes), sugary desserts, cake icing, fruit snacks, South Beach oatmeal cookies, Rice Krispies Treats, Lifesavers, jelly beans, candy corn, Dots, soft peppermints, Smarties, small Snickers bars, and other sugar-filled things. Gladys Dull almost always drinks orange juice when she's low, although she also carries wrapped candy in her purse when she goes out. She says, "If I only had a dollar for every orange I've drunk as juice in my life, I'd be rich!" For her, juice works as fast as anything.

What you treat yourself with may also need to vary with the circumstances. If you're only slightly low, you may just need a glucose tablet or two. If you're low and likely to keep dropping from whatever insulin you have on board, then you may benefit by taking in some food or a drink with greater staying power, something with some fat or protein to go with the carbs, like peanut butter crackers or Balance Bars. Milk is additionally a good treatment option for that reason, since one serving contains seven to eight grams of protein, along with some fat depending on what type you're drinking. Skim milk works pretty well, but at least one study showed that for prevention of lows following exercise, whole milk is much more effective than skim or even sports drinks (likely because of the extra fat in it).

Gerald Cleveland prefers Quaker Oats Chewy Granola Bars or Nature Valley Trail Mix Granola Bars, while Al Lewis prefers Gatorade (made from powder at twice the normal concentration). For longer-term prevention of lows, Al will often eat bread with jam or a muffin. Carolyn Balcom uses glucose tablets followed by some juice if her blood sugar is below 55 mg/dl, but if it's a little higher and she still needs something else, she eats grapes. "I carry a little dish of red, purple, or black grapes around with me in my purse." Has grapes in purse, will travel? Now, there's a woman who loves her grapes.

AND THE LAST ONE TO THE FINISH LINE IS . . . JUICE?

Skim milk, orange juice, and sugary drinks were the usual recommended treatments for low blood sugar reactions from years ago. Over the years, Dr. Sheri has gravitated to using glucose tablets for the first-line treatment of lows because, for her, they always seem to have the most rapid effect. We now know a lot more about the glycemic effects of foods than we used to, and with the glycemic index in mind, it also makes sense that glucose would work most rapidly. The glycemic index (GI) for glucose is ranked 100, with table sugar at 68, juices ranging from 40 for apple to 48 for grapefruit and 57 for orange, regular sodas at 63, and skim milk ranking only 32. (As an aside, only a few foods have a GI higher than straight glucose, such as the cookies and cream Clif Bar and Desiree potatoes from Australia that have been peeled and boiled for 35 minutes, both of which have a GI of 101, along with select others that range up to 104.)

With these facts in mind, Dr. Sheri got her nondiabetic oldest son, Alex, interested in doing his seventh grade science fair project on the differences in the rate of absorption and peak glucose increase caused by consuming various sugars. (There's nothing like having a mother who's a diabetes researcher, is there?) Glucose is a simple sugar ($C_6H_{12}O_6$), as is fructose (fruit sugar). The sugar in milk, lactose, is actually made of one galactose sugar (the third simple kind) and one glucose, while table sugar (sucrose) is half glucose, half fructose. In theory, then, glucose should have the fastest effect because it's already in the form your body needs to raise blood sugars. Conversely, the fructose in fruit and table sugar have to be converted to glucose through enzymatic reactions in the body, as does the galactose that makes up half of milk sugar.

Although oral glucose testing usually involves consuming seventy-five grams of carbs, with self-preservation in mind, Dr. Sheri decided that fifteen grams of carbs from the various sugars would be enough to test the glycemic effects on herself and her son (bless his heart—he did all the finger sticking every ten minutes for an hour for twelve trials as well, but we left his results out), and an hour would be long enough to study the resulting rise (since you'd hope your blood sugars would be back to normal in much less than sixty minutes). The following graphs of Alex's testing results on his diabetic mother are the average of three trials for each sugar done on separate days prior to her taking any rapid-acting insulin in the morning, so only her basal dose of Lantus was on board during the tests.

As you can see, glucose and sucrose were surprisingly similar in their effects, causing a significant rise in her blood sugars in ten to twenty minutes, while skim milk only lagged behind in how rapidly it raised blood sugars. The milk had a more lasting effect, though, and caused a more extended rise by fifty minutes afterward, likely due to its protein content. The juice (grapefruit with pure fructose and no added high-fructose corn syrup) lagged severely behind the others, and never reached close to the same levels, making it the least effective rapid treatment for hypoglycemia. Even though this study design had its limitations, Dick Bernstein would likely agree with the results, as he says, "O.J. is too slow to be good for treating lows." By way of comparison, in 12-year-old Alex (whose graph is not shown), glucose tablets made his blood sugar rise 70 mg/dl in the first half hour, but then it came right back down within the hour. None of the other three sugars caused more than a temporary 20 to 30 mg/dl increase.

DR. SHERI'S GLYCEMIC RESPONSES TO FIFTEEN GRAMS OF EACH TYPE OF SUGAR

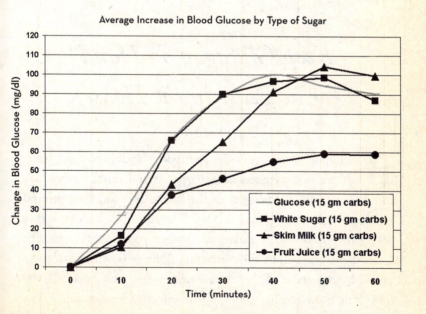

Average Increase in Blood Glucose by Type of Sugar

It may seem like common sense, but another secret is to always make certain that you carry something with you to treat your lows. More times than we can remember, we have heard stories of people with diabetes who just stepped out of the house and forgot the bring something with them, and then had a bad low blood sugar reaction. Dr. Sheri remembers the story of one hard-training triathlete who always carried something with her during her long, strenuous workouts, but would go out to walk the dog without taking anything with her and have her blood sugars drop like a rock. (Perhaps for her, taking the dog out just didn't seem like enough exercise to cause a low blood sugar, but believe us, it can.) The motto for treating lows, then, should probably be the following: "Always be prepared."

❧ 17 ❧

Keep Glucagon on Hand (or at Least in the House)

Bad hypoglycemic episodes that you're unable to treat yourself are best avoided all at costs. If you can't, though, it's important to have glucagon in the house and someone around who knows how to give it to you. Glucagon is a hormone that your pancreas normally makes, even when you have diabetes. It's formed and released by the pancreatic alpha cells, which are unaffected by the onset of the disease even when your beta cells are lost. This hormone has the opposite effect of insulin, and when your liver is exposed to it, this glucose-regulating organ is stimulated to release more glucose into your bloodstream.

Glucagon is available as a prescribed emergency kit that can be stored at room temperature or in the refrigerator and is stable for several years after purchase. It contains a freeze-dried version of it that must be mixed with glycerin in solution and then injected into your muscle (front of thighs or upper arm) or into the skin like insulin injections—either way works. Injecting glucagon is the fastest way to raise a low blood sugar, but someone who has been trained to mix and inject it needs to be available to give it to you. When you resist treatment for a low, become unconscious, or have seizures from a bad low, glucagon can be used to rapidly raise your blood sugar. You can also self-inject it when you're ill or nauseated and can't eat anything to treat a low blood sugar. A full dose (usually 1 mg) is appropriate for a 200-pound person, but if you weigh 150 pounds or less, a half dose is sufficient, and giving more is likely to cause severe nausea. If someone gives you glucagon when you're unconscious, you may not come out of it fully for ten to fifteen minutes, and then you may feel very nauseated for a period of time afterward (even after getting a smaller dose). Lethargy and seeming "out of it" for a while afterward are also common, but if these symptoms persist, you may need to be taken to the emergency room.

Before glucagon was evenly widely available, Dee Brehm got some and gave it to her husband to keep handy so that he would be ready to treat her with it, if needed. For Jane Dohrmann, her recent problems with bad hypoglycemic events have made it important for her to keep glucagon in her house. "My son is not good at giving me glucagon," she says, "but my husband is." One time she knew a low was coming on (she had checked and was 54 mg/dl) and was on her way downstairs to get some milk. She made it there, had a sip of milk, but never got the crackers she was going to eat opened up. She woke up with paramedics all around her that fortunately her son had called. An injection of glucagon administered by her husband in that situation (if he had been at home instead of just her son) would have prevented the need for a 911 call and brought her out of her low blood sugar reaction sooner.

Severe low blood sugar reactions that are not detected or treated with glucagon can be fatal, so it's important that you have someone check on you from time to time if you live alone. Also, let others know where you keep the glucagon and train them on how to inject you with glucagon if the need arises. The sooner your low is treated, the better. Severe hypoglycemic comas actually cause some of the nerve cells in your brain to die, which can lead to impairment of cognitive abilities following such an episode. Apparently, getting a dose of pyruvate (a metabolite that is produced from glucose) within three hours may help since, for some reason, glucose-starved brain cells apparently have a hard time using glucose after a bad low, but pyruvate can provide them with an alternate fuel that they can use.

18

Find the Right Doctor (and a Diabetes Educator, Too)

If you want to do well with your diabetes over the long haul, find a really good doctor or medical support team. They should be up-to-date on the latest research, technologies, medications, and more. If you question your doctor's judgment, seek out a second opinion about your diabetes care, and switch doctors if you need to in order to find someone who is more knowledgeable. In theory, you should not know more about diabetes and its appropriate care than your doctor, although Gerald Cleveland's doctor told him that Gerald is a "student of diabetes," who knows more about it than his own doctor does. (That's what living with diabetes for 75 years can do for you.)

The Joslin Diabetes Center has long been known for its high standing in cutting-edge diabetes care. Dr. Steve did a fellowship there after receiving his medical training, and Dr. Sheri was a patient there for a week when she was 13 and visiting Boston for a month one summer. At the time, she wasn't happy about going, as her father had decided to "incarcerate" her there without any advance warning. In retrospect, though, she realizes that it was one of the most beneficial experiences of her young life with diabetes (9 year's worth already at that point).

Other diabetes survivors have also benefited from their Joslin Center experiences. For instance, Patty Schaeffer's cousin, Kent, developed diabetes, and his father (her uncle) looked for the best place to send him for medical care. Patty had already had diabetes for over 7 years at the point but had not been to the Joslin for care. After Kent came back from his visit there, his mother was so impressed by the positive changes in his physical health that, unbeknownst to Patty, her aunt arranged for her to go there for a week of training as well. Patty remembers, "I was in class and got called down to the principal's office. I wondered what I'd done wrong! When I got there, my mother and Aunt Gladys were there to take me to Long Island and then to Boston to the Joslin Center." Her first diabetes mentor was her doctor there, and after a successful first visit, she went back periodically over the years. Freddi Fredrickson, who lives in Southern California, actually lived in Boston near the Joslin Center when she was diagnosed in 1961. "I went to a week program there," she recalls, "and I really got a good education from the start." Natalie Saunders was similarly impressed with all Joslin had to offer back when information about diabetes was not abundant, and she went there several times to learn more about carbohydrate and food exchanges, among other things.

FINDING A DIABETES EDUCATOR—LIKELY ONE OF THE MOST VITAL RELATIONSHIPS YOU WILL HAVE

Even if you only have access to a good diabetes educator, this association can serve you well. Many of them are living with diabetes themselves, which just increases their awareness of the possible problems you can encounter and how to overcome them. An excellent place to turn to find one if you don't have access in your area is online diabetes education resources. For example, located in Wynnewood, Pennsylvania, founded and run by Gary Scheiner, MS, who got his diabetes training at the renowned Joslin Diabetes Center, Integrated Diabetes Services boasts a team of educators to provide personal diabetes coaching and counseling from afar via Internet (www.integratedservices.com) and telephone (877-SELF-MGT). You can find other similarly beneficial resources on the Internet as well, including on the Web site of the American Association of Diabetes Educators (found at www.aadenet.org), which has a diabetes educator locator by city and state. Alternately, you can call them toll-free to be directed to an educator in your area at (800) 338-3633.

Alternately, Gladys Dull benefited from her early care and education at the Mayo Clinic in Rochester, Minnesota. "I was just fortunate that my parents could take me there from North Dakota when I was first diagnosed," she says. Since that initial visit in 1924, she has been back many times, including once when her husband was overseas during WWII.

Generally, a diabetes specialist or an endocrinologist will be able to give you the best care, and many long-living people with diabetes, like Carol Sessions, Karen Poenisch, Bernadette McIntyre, and Blondie Fram, advise that you find a good endocrinologist. "You have to go to the right kind of doctor—not to an internist who doesn't know anything about counting carbs," agrees Patricia La France-Wolf. She also acknowledges, however, that you have to have good medical coverage to deal effectively with your diabetes medical care. She admits to being lucky enough that her medical coverage has allowed her to pick her own doctors over the years. For Ron DeNunzio, the key is "to find a doctor that will listen to you as a person, will understand your needs and wants, and is willing to grow with you." Finding a good diabetes doctor in all areas of the country (and world) is not necessarily an easy task, but it is one that is likely to benefit you immensely. Don Gifford asserts that finding the best medical care that you can possibly get is important, and as a University of Maryland law professor, he contends that most of the best medical practices are located in urban centers, particularly teaching hospitals. In fact, he initially moved to Maryland to get better eye care. "The quality of health care varies widely," he states unequivocally. Luckily for Peter Gariti, he learned the value of having an endocrinologist when his first employer in Chicago connected him up with one locally at Northwestern Medical School. "I think it's important that people get treated by an endocrinologist, a diabetes specialist," he says. "I had other doctors when my job moved me around, but they didn't know as much. General practitioners know very little about diabetes, and internists only know some. Get to a specialist if you can."

Because of her medical experiences, Mary Sue Rubin also advises people to search out the best medical team they can find. For doctors to work for her, they have to be willing to try things her way instead of just their own, and she really believed you have to coordinate all your care yourself. Over the years, she has run across a lot of ignorance in the general medical community regarding diabetes, which should be a warning to you to seek more specialized care. For instance, when she was in the hospital for pneumonia, the doctor asked her about her insulin regimen. When she told him she was using Regular insulin and a longer-acting one, he told her that both insulins were "the same." On her next admission, a hospital nutritionist asked her if she eats lunch meat—and that was after Mary Sue had already told the woman that she's a vegetarian. Experiences like these only made her realize how much she needs to be in control of her own health.

Marialice Kern agrees, saying that everyone should seek out a good physician who is on top of research and who will treat you like the educated person that you have become. For Jessica Ching, it's all about matching yourself to your doctor. "If your doctor isn't right for you, it won't work," she says. Matt Besley feels lucky that his father sent him to see a doctor who had type 1 diabetes himself. This doctor gave Matt some good advice early on, telling him, "Ultimately, you're the one in control of this disease and the one to decide what to do." To this day, Matt realizes the value of finding a really good doctor. He advises people, "Be around doctors, different ones, to see who's good and who's not. Look out for yourself. Find someone who's interested in new therapies and technologies." For others, including Matthew Lore from New York, the publisher of this book (who has had type 1 diabetes for more than a decade), finding a doctor that will make enough time to listen to them during office visits is most important. Matthew states, "My doctor needs to have or make the time to let me give a brief rundown of what's going on and any changes or problems. I know they're under tremendous pressure from insurance companies to get patients in and out in less than ten to fifteen minutes, but a willingness to listen (and then, of course, respond accordingly) *and* to hear me as an individual, and not a 'type,' is for me the first and most critical, nonnegotiable requirement I have in a doctor."

As mentioned, Dr. Steve is a strong advocate for people taking control of their own health and their diabetes, and to that end, he is constantly trying to educate people whenever and wherever the opportunity arises. "I met him in 1989 at the VA Hospital in San Diego," Will Speer, Sr., says about Dr. Steve. "He heard me asking another doctor for information, and he asked if I'd like to talk. He got me on an insulin pump—I was the first vet at Navy Hospital with one back then—and he helped me in other ways. I attribute still being alive to him." Vena Petrotta, who has considered her diabetes to be brittle for close to the past sixty years, also thinks it's important to go to your doctor or an emergency room at the first sign of trouble, especially for bad hypoglycemia or diabetic ketoacidosis (DKA). "I have always kept in close contact with my doctors," she says.

Even Robert Mandell, an 84-year-old resident of Richmond, Virginia, who has been living with type 2 diabetes for more than four decades, believes that seeing a doctor regularly is one of the secrets to his longevity with diabetes. If you can afford to, you may want to consider following his advice: "The VA Hospital will only allow me to see a doctor twice a year, so I see a private physician for my diabetes every three months." He has also benefited from getting occasional free advice from his son, Barry Mandell, MD, an ophthalmologist specializing in retinal problems in Virginia Beach, Virginia, who has also helped his mother-in-law, Natalie Saunders, control her retinopathy. Blondie Fram, who has had type 2 diabetes at least as long as Robert, agrees with him. "Just listen to your doctor," she advises, "and go see an endocrinologist, not just an ordinary doctor." She too has benefited from good medical support by a related medical doctor, her son-in-law, Aaron Vinik, MD, PhD, a world-renowned diabetic neuropathy specialist in Norfolk, Virginia.

AL LEWIS, AGE 73, LIVING WITH TYPE 1 DIABETES FOR 69 YEARS

If you know Al Lewis, a resident of Vancouver, BC, you will understand why he waited to start using an insulin pump until there was a waterproof model available (1997): His whole life has revolved around water, one way or another. He fished commercially off the coast of California when he was only 12 years old, and despite having diabetes since the age of 4, he would be out at sea for days at a time (with only a partner and without his parents). "I think it was harder on my parents than it was on me," he reminisces. "My mom used to get up at 2:00 AM to make me breakfast before I would go out fishing, and she told me later that she would cry after I left." He had just become a teenager when he got a certificate from the United States Power Squadron for completing its small boat course, making him at that time the youngest person to ever complete it.

After a three-year foray into forestry at the start of college, he soon found himself drawn to the study of oceanography instead (big surprise there). In both his undergraduate and master's degree studies, he was on the swim team and lettered at both levels. His PhD degree research at the University of Hawaii involved skin diving and some scuba diving. Until just recently, he was still involved in swimming competitively at the master's level (defined as age 25 and older for swimming).

An emeritus professor of oceanography at the University of British Columbia, Al is convinced that all of his activity has played a large role in his diabetes longevity—close to 70 years already—and his lack of any major diabetes-related health problems. Fear of complications is a driving motivation to take care of himself, though. "I think one secret of longevity with diabetes is to be very competitive with yourself," he says, recalling that he was even more competitive with himself than with other swimmers he swam against over the years. "I think it's key to being successful with diabetes."

You can tell that Al is a dedicated swimmer when you hear about some of the things he has done. For example, he once contacted a swimming outfitter in Portland, Oregon, to see if they could make a suit that could be worn in a swimming pool and hold an insulin pump (the waterproof kind, of course). He had been wearing a fanny pack with his pump inside—both for safety when he was out at sea as an oceanographer and also while swimming. In the end, they couldn't come up with anything innovative for him, so he just swims in a triathlete full-body suit with his insulin pump tucked inside.

Some recent back problems have propelled Al out of the pool and into the gym for weight workouts, but he continues to commute to campus and back by bicycle. Given his lifetime of physical activity, it is highly unlikely that he will let anything stop him now, especially not a small thing like diabetes.

PART FOUR

Dietary Secrets

19

Watch Your Diet, and Watch It Good

All long-living diabetes survivors agree that eating a healthy diet is as important as any other aspect of their success with diabetes. They were originally taught to use the diabetic exchange diet, which promoted a balanced intake of carbohydrates, fat, and protein for meals and snacks—with more emphasis placed sometimes on low carbs and other times on low fat intake. Both Karen Poenisch and Dr. Sheri vividly remember the vegetable exchanges, though, with group A and B vegetables (Karen's memory) and 3 percent and 6 percent veggies (Dr. Sheri's memorized categories). Regardless of the approach, the idea was that some vegetables are lower in carbs (like lettuce, green beans, broccoli, cauliflower, and more), while others, like potatoes, sweet potatoes, green peas, corn, and carrots, were starchier and had to be watched more closely.

To this day (almost 40 years later), Dr. Sheri has these categories of veggies in the back of her mind when she chooses the daily vegetables for her family's dinner. She says, "Only the lower-carb ones count as a true vegetable as far as I'm concerned, and they're the ones I eat in the largest quantity. The starchy ones count towards my carbohydrate and insulin intake, and I limit my intake of those." She also limits her intake of anything with a higher glycemic effect—like white-flour products, breads, pizza, and most sweets—but also closely watches overall intake of carbohydrate-rich foods that are absorbed more slowly, such as brown rice, sweet potatoes, pasta, legumes, and fruits. Likewise, Dr. Steve started out using the exchange system, and he still doesn't do any official carb counting, although he does guesstimate his premeal boluses with a correction factor of approximately one unit of insulin for every forty grams of carbs. (Your own carb ratio may vary from this one. For instance, Dr. Sheri's is closer to one unit for every fifteen grams, but in the morning it's more like ten grams.)

Jane Dohrmann also remembers starting out with an exchange diet over 40 years ago. As for a specific diet back when she was first diagnosed, she recalls, "I'm not sure that I had recommendations for a diet, but I did have 'instructions' for a 1,800 calorie diet that I followed to the letter using the exchange system." In comparing those earlier days with her diet today, she says, "People have no idea how very fortunate they are today that foods are so much more available for those of us with diabetes. There are far more healthy foods, the food labels are better, and the artificial sweeteners are much more palatable. And there's sugar-free chocolate pudding!" She continues to watch her intake of carbs and sugar to this day but gives herself a little more freedom since she can bolus for her carbs and usually has no problems doing so.

"Managing your diet is important," agrees Patricia La France-Wolf. "You can't just go pig out on everything." She started out on a low carbohydrate, high fat diet almost 63 years ago, and she still limits her carbohydrate intake to less than eighty grams a day.

"I eat almost everything I want to eat, but I just don't eat large amounts." Similarly, one of Freddi Fredrickson's secrets of longevity with diabetes is not to eat a lot of carbohydrates. "I just eat enough, but not too much!" she says. Early in her years with diabetes, her diet was a lot more inconsistent, and without a blood glucose meter, her blood sugars were a lot harder to control, given her very inconsistent eating patterns. Vena Petrotta's attitude is similar. "Sometimes eating carbs is just not worth it," she remarks. "I watch my fat intake, too."

Most of the longest-living people with diabetes have generally weighed out all their food at some point in their lives, along with controlling their portion sizes and keeping meticulous food records of everything they ate or drank. For years, Gladys Dull weighed out all of her food, but now she can usually guess a food's weight without using a scale due to her long experience with doing so; she also varies her diet very little and has consistent eating times. Likewise, Dee Brehm's secret for success with diabetes centers around measuring everything for the 58 years. "I measure everything—my food, my blood glucose, and my blood pressure—and I write everything down. I have only missed one time in the last 58 years." In addition, she limits her carbohydrate intake to twenty-five to thirty grams at each meal, for which she takes a set dose of insulin.

Carolyn Balcom also finds that her discipline is one of her secrets for taking care of herself. Like Dee Brehm, she also has been thorough in her record keeping over 43 years of living with diabetes. "I keep records of not only my blood sugars and insulin, but also my activity and the foods that I eat," she says. "For many years, I used small spiral notebooks for this, but now I use the ezManager program from Animas (an insulin pump company). I have this program on my Palm Pilot, and I find it very helpful. It has a good food database to which I have added many other of my own with the nutrition info from food labels." She adds, "I can download the records to my computer and print out what I need. It helps me and my endocrinologist." (As an aside, the ezManager software allows users to create and store an individualized food database right on their Animas IR 1250 pump, as does their newer 2020 that allows storage of 500 chosen items. See more on insulin pumps and their features in Secret 32). The primary benefit of such meticulous record keeping is being able to see how various foods and activities affect your blood sugar, along with finding trends (such as always running high at a particular time of day) that allow you to make adjustments to your medications or dietary regimens.

When it comes to diabetes control and good health, dietary fiber intake is important as well. Karen Poenisch advises eating low fat and not overloading on the carbs, unless they're full of fiber—like popcorn, most veggies, and beans. In addition, she uses a fiber supplement, Fibersure, which she says really helps with her blood sugar control. "It's hard to take in the recommended twenty-five to thirty grams of fiber every day," she says, "so I supplement to make sure I get them." She focuses on taking in whole grains and other fiber-rich foods. Similarly, John Rodosevich really likes to eat high-fiber fruits, like pears. "I hardly have to take any insulin for them because of the fiber," he says. Bernadette McIntyre also advocates eating more fruits and vegetables, along with a limited amount of carbs. She has found the Weight Watchers Diet to be an effective one in helping her prevent weight gain (and control her diabetes), largely because of its high fiber content and plentiful intake of water.

Most people with diabetes admit that initially following dietary guidelines of any sort has led them to have a healthier diet in general. For example, Rich Humphreys makes his own bread using whole wheat and almond flour, and he adds lots of almonds, walnuts, and raisins to it. He eats plenty of veggies and lots of soups. "I was brought up on a healthy diet," he states simply. Similarly, Mary Sue Rubin continues to eat a very healthy, organic diet, with no red meat or pork, lots of fruits and veggies, whole grains, no preservatives, and only occasional chocolate. "I grew up eating healthy food throughout my childhood, too," she remarks. So did Bernadette McIntyre. "When I was young, we ate baked and boiled foods, not fried. Our eating didn't change that much after I got diabetes, except for not taking any more trips to the penny store for candy." Dr. Sheri also remembers that her mother changed the whole family's diet to match the American Diabetes Association's exchange diet at the time (1968), and to this day, she feels she eats a healthier diet because of the eating habits that she established in childhood.

Likewise, Carolyn Balcom made a decision early on in her life with diabetes to be careful about what she ate. Immediately after she was found to have sugar in her urine and her diabetes was diagnosed, the then 29-year-old bought and ate a Hershey bar. "My thought was that this was the last one I would ever eat, and it has been—except for the sugar-free kind. My husband thinks that this helped me say good-bye to sweets," she recalls. (Many of the rest of us still eat regular chocolate to this day, though, but just in moderation, particularly since dark chocolate is especially packed full of healthy phytonutrients and antioxidants.)

It also used to be much harder to find many foods that were prepared with diabetic individuals with mind, such as canned fruits that weren't packed in heavy syrup. Years ago, though, Jim Arthur's parents found canned fruit packed in water in Chicago (which was pretty far from where he lived), and they used to buy cases of it for him during the winter. "It was pretty tasteless," he recalls, "but it was better than no fruit at all during the winter." He still eats a healthy, low-fat diet that includes lots of veggies, fish, lots of salads, and only significant carbs on special occasions (for which he takes more insulin).

GETTING YOURSELF MORE NUTRITION SAVVY (WITH ONLINE TOOLS AND RESOURCES)

Nutrition Analysis Tools and System (NATS 2.0) (online nutritional analysis): http://nat.crgq.com/index2.html

Nutrition Facts and Calorie Counter (single foods analyses and calorie counter): www.nutritiondata.com

Eating Well Do-It-Yourself Nutrition Analysis Tool (full nutrition analysis and calorie counts by single ingredient, brand-name foods, and restaurant-chain meals): www.eatingwell.com/health_diet/nutrition_tools/diy_nutrition_analysis.html

USDA National Nutrient Database (searchable nutritional content of individual foods): www.nal.usda.gov/fnic/foodcomp/search or www.ars.usda.gov/main/site_main.htm?modecode=12354500 or www.ars.usda.gov/Services/docs.htm?docid=8964

Tufts University Health & Nutrition Letter (good source of updated nutritional information): http://healthletter.tufts.edu

Tufts University Nutrition Resources (links): http://hnrc.tufts.edu/resources/nutrition.shtml

Center for Science in the Public Interest (Nutrition Action health letter and more): www.cspinet.org

USDA Center for Nutrition Policy and Promotion (links to dietary guidelines and new food guide pyramid): www.cnpp.usda.gov

USDA Food Guide Pyramid (latest recommendations): www.mypyramid.gov

Nutrition.gov (dietary guidelines and supplement facts): www.nutrition.gov

CDC Division of Nutrition and Physical Activity (nutritional education resources): www.cdc.gov/nccdphp/dnpa

Center for Food Safety and Applied Nutrition (links to nutrition-related information): www.cfsan.fda.gov

Fruits and Veggies Matter (a government site): www.fruitsandveggiesmatter.gov or www.5aday.gov

Not everyone does anything remarkable with his or her diet, though. Grant McArthur eats about 2,400 calories a day, but he says, "I've been at it so long that I know how much insulin I need for my food." Peter Gariti doesn't officially carb count, but he says he has a rough idea of the amount of insulin he needs to cover anything he eats, and he watches his carb intake. Chuck Eichten admits the same thing. "I don't count carbs, but I do have a sense of what effects certain foods will have," he says. He eats a well-rounded diet with fish as his main protein intake, but he especially watches the quantity of foods he eats. For the occasional cookie or dessert, he takes an extra bolus of insulin if he needs to, but usually it just fits in with his normal food intake. Paul McGuigan doesn't follow any special diet either, but he just covers what he eats with insulin, which he says works for him. Admittedly, developing the knowledge to "know" how much to give is a combination of trial-and-error and instinct.

Likewise, Natalie Saunders never eats too many carbs at one time, and she limits her fruit intake to one piece a day and pizza to about once a month. Not all fruits are taboo for people with diabetes, though, and the health benefits of eating more may outweigh any diabetic concerns. Many have lots of fiber and are absorbed slowly enough to not cause much of a spike in blood glucose levels. For instance, almost all types of berries (strawberries, blueberries, raspberries, blackberries, cranberries, etc.) have a low glycemic effect and not much carbohydrates for a typical serving. For a list of the glycemic rankings of the rest of the fruit world, refer to the table that appears later in this secret. She's right to avoid eating much pizza, however, as it is well known to raise blood glucose levels for hours after you eat it.

Will Speer, Sr., admits to being a meat-and-potatoes person and says his diet has not changed much in the past 39 years with diabetes. "I don't count or limit my carbs," he says. "I just use a sliding scale, and I know how much insulin I need to bolus with for what I eat." He does, however, credit his wife with providing him with a consistent diet of three meals a day at the same times. It's likely that having his life well regulated in this way has helped him maintain control over his blood sugars. Similarly, Matt Besley admits to limiting his carb intake, eating lots of protein, and many fruits and vegetables. "I consistently eat the same foods," he says, "because that makes it easier to predict what their effect will be."

On the other hand, Blondie Fram is extremely careful with her food intake to control her type 2 diabetes. "I have learned to do without a lot of things," she says. "It really doesn't worry me. I eat everything, but just not anything with added sugar. My diet is balanced—with plenty of salad, green vegetables, carbs, and protein—but I don't eat large quantities." To control his type 2 diabetes for the past 40 years, Robert Mandell also realizes the importance of adhering to your diet. "Don't starve yourself," he advises, "but just know what to eat." Like Blondie, he eats almost everything, but only in limited quantities, such as no more than small portions of pasta in the evenings and only half of a baked potato. He also limits his intake of bread and eats only sugar-free desserts. In addition, he eats plenty of salads, beans, fish, and soup.

So, it appears that for most long-time diabetic survivors, limiting intake of carbs (but not eliminating them altogether) has proven to be an important part of their diabetes control. A newer concept than using exchanges is the related idea of categorizing carbohydrates by both the rapidity that they're turned into glucose (their glycemic index, or GI) and their total quantity of carbohydrate per serving (glycemic load, or GL). All of the GI values are derived from clinical studies of people with and without diabetes. For the few diabetic individuals who have been studied, their blood glucose responses to more rapidly absorbed carbohydrates have been exaggerated. Thus, if you have to give insulin to try to match the rise in blood glucose, you're insulin resistant, or your body fails to release enough insulin quickly in response to food intake (which is the case for most individuals with type 2 diabetes), then your blood sugars are likely to spike even higher and more rapidly than predicted by a food's GI. As for GL, it represents the product of food's GI and its total available carbohydrate content (with fiber excluded) in a "typical" serving. Since everyone with diabetes has trouble with having insulin peak at just the right time to cover the blood glucose spikes resulting from high-GI and high-GL food intake, the best way to effectively manage your diabetes is to regulate both, which you can do by avoiding overloading your diet with carbohydrates, particularly ones with higher GI values.

When selecting which foods to eat, take into account the glycemic effect, the total carbohydrate content, and the nutrient density of your meals and snacks. It's best to limit your intake of foods with both a high or medium GI value and a high GL (as listed in the box that follows), unless you're using the carbs to treat or prevent hypoglycemia, particularly during exercise. Any carbohydrate-rich meal (i.e., one with an overall high GL) will require more insulin for your body to process it, but at least if the GI value is lower (such as when fiber content is high), you'll have a less immediate rise in your blood sugars. Therefore, either the insulin you give will be absorbed quickly enough to cover the rise more effectively for such foods (if you give insulin), or your body's inability to release a large amount of insulin at once will be less critical.

An alternative strategy that some insulin users employ for carbohydrate intake is "pre-bolusing," or giving their insulin from ten to thirty minutes before they start eating so that more of it is available by the time the glucose from the carbs hits the bloodstream. (See Secret 31 to learn more about the time it takes different insulins to peak.) Doing so does more effectively control

GLYCEMIC INDEX (PER FIFTY GRAMS OF AVAILABLE CARBOHYDRATE) AN[D] GLYCEMIC LOAD (PER "TYPICAL" SERVING) (GI, GL)

	Low GI (0 to 55)	Medium GI (56 to 69)	High GI (70 to 100)
LOW GL (< 10)	Apples (38,6)	Apricots (57,5)	Bread, white flour (70,10)
	Beans, baked (48,7)	Beets (64,5)	Bread, whole-wheat (71,9)
	Beans, kidney (28,7)	Bread, 7-grain (55,8)	Glucose (99,10)
	Beans, pinto (39,10)	Cantaloupe (65,4)	Popcorn (72,8)
	Bread, whole-grain (51,7)	Honey (55,10)	Watermelon (72,4)
	Carrots (47,3)	Ice cream, regular (61,8)	
	Cereal, All-Bran (42,9)	Peaches, canned in heavy syrup (55,9)	
	Chickpeas (28,8)	Pineapple (59,7)	
	Cookie, oatmeal (54,9)	Sugar, white (68,7)	
	Corn, sweet (54,9)		
	Fructose sweetener (20,2)		
	Grapefruit (25,3)		
	Grapes (46,8)		
	Ice cream, low-fat (43,5)		
	Ice cream, premium (38,4)		
	Juice, carrot (43,10)		
	Juice, tomato (38,4)		
	Lentils, red (26,5)		
	M&M's, peanut (33,6)		
	Milk, skim (32,4)		
	Milk, soy (42,7)		
	Milk, whole (40,3)		
	Oranges (42,5)		
	Peaches (42,5)		
	Peaches, canned in juice (38,9)		
	Peanuts (14,1)		
	Pears (38,4)		
	Peas, green (48,3)		
	Prunes (29,10)		
	Strawberries (40,1)		
	Tortellini, cheese (50,10)		
	Yogurt, low-fat (27,7)		
	Yogurt, nonfat, artificially sweetened (24,3)		

	Low GI (0 to 55)	Medium GI (56 to 69)	High GI (70 to 100)
DIUM

TO 19) | Bananas (52,12)
Barley, pearled (25,11)
Beans, navy (38,12)
Bread, sourdough wheat (54,15)
Buckwheat (54,16)
Cookie bar, Twix (44,17)
Corn, sweet (53,17)
Juice, apple (40,12)
Juice, grapefruit (48,11)
Juice, orange (50,12)
Juice, pineapple (46,16)
Pasta, fettuccine (40,18)
Ravioli, meat (39,15)
Rice, parboiled (47,17) | Cake, angel food (67,19)
Cereal, Life (66,16)
Cereal, Raisin Bran (61,12)
Cereal, Special K (69,14)
Croissant (67,17)
Juice, orange (57,15)
Muffin, bran (60,15)
Oatmeal, old-fashioned (58,13)
Oatmeal, quick (66,17)
Pizza, cheese (60,16)
Potatoes, new (57,12)
Potatoes, sweet (61,17)
Rice, brown, boiled (55,18)
Rice, wild (57,18) | Doughnut, cake-type (76,17)
Cereal, Cheerios (74,15)
Cereal, Grape Nuts (75,16)
Cereal, shredded wheat (75,15)
Cereal, Total (76,17)
Crackers, soda (74,12)
Gatorade, 12 oz. (78,17)
Potatoes, mashed (85,17)
Pretzels (83,16)
Muffin, English (77,11)
Rice cakes, puffed (78, 17)
Wafers, vanilla (77,14) |

	Low GI (0 to 55)	Medium GI (56 to 69)	High GI (70 to 100)
H GL

) | Pasta, linguine (46,22)
Pasta, macaroni (47,23)
Pasta, spaghetti (44,21) | Candy bar, Mars (65,26)
Candy bar, Snickers (68,23)
Coca-Cola, 12-oz. can (63,23)
Cranberry juice cocktail (68,24)
Couscous (65,23)
Kudos, whole-grain bar, chocolate chip (62,20)
Macaroni and cheese, boxed (64,32)
Power Bar (56,24)
Raisins (64,28)
Rice, white, boiled (64,23) | Bagel, white flour (72,25)
Candy, Skittles (70,32)
Cereal, cornflakes (92,24)
Cereal, Golden Grahams (71,18)
Cereal, Krispix (87,22)
Cereal, Rice Krispies (82,22)
French fries (75,22)
Fruit bars, strawberry (90,23)
Fruit Roll-Ups (99,24)
Jelly beans (78,22)
Potato, baked russet (85,26)
Pop-Tart, double chocolate (70,24) |

after-meal peaks most of the time, but the downside is that if the GI of what you've eaten is low enough, your insulin may outpace your food, making you end up hypoglycemic. You also are held to eating a certain amount of carbohydrate for the insulin you've already given. One more strategy is to split your dose, as long as you don't mind multiple injections or extra boluses. For instance, Dr. Sheri oftentimes gives half of the insulin she expects to need awhile before she starts eating, and then she gives the rest of what she actually needs for the carbs she has eaten. If the majority of the carbs you're eating is composed of nonstarchy vegetables and low GI fruits, though, you may not benefit from giving most of your insulin that far in advance.

🦋 20 🦋

Count Your Carbs

As mentioned, most people who have lived with diabetes for longer than 20 years started out on the American Diabetes Association's diabetes exchange diet that balanced the intake of specific portions ("exchanges") of carbs, fats, and protein, before evolving into now focusing on carbohydrate counting since the arrival of blood glucose meters on the scene. Because the majority of insulin (beyond basal needs) is given to cover your carbohydrate intake, knowing how many grams you are eating and how much insulin you usually need for a certain number of grams becomes critical to maintaining good control. Studies have shown that consistency in the amount and source of carbohydrate intake from day to day is associated with improved blood glucose control in people with type 1 diabetes. However, such findings may not be as relevant to you if you're on intensified insulin therapy and adjust your insulin doses based on your actual carbohydrate intake at each meal.

If you've been diagnosed with diabetes in the past decade, you likely have simply been taught how to count carbs (without any importance attributed to their GI) and balance them out with the right amount of rapid-acting insulin to cover them, but to do so you must be taking insulin specifically for meals and snacks. Larry Verity used to count calories, not just carbs, but most of what he was eating was carbs, so now he just counts them, although he still eats somewhere in the range of 1,600 to 2,000 calories daily. Even most old-timers have learned to keep track of their carbohydrate intake and adjust their insulin doses accordingly, although many would agree with Marialice Kern, who says, "Carb counting is not an easy thing." To be really accurate, your counting would likely require you to read food labels and then measure out everything that you're eating. Doing so is often very challenging—and sometimes nearly impossible—for most foods cooked at home from scratch, restaurant foods (for which there usually aren't carb contents or measuring devices available), and combination foods like pizza.

For Patty Schaeffer, counting carbs has worked well, though. "I have always had severe insulin reactions that have been constant—a 'normal' part of my life. Counting carbs has really simplified things. Since right before I went on a pump in 2000, my bad lows have stopped. I think the credit really goes to having a better judgment of my food." Along similar lines, Carolyn Balcom started carb counting when she first went on a basal insulin/rapid-acting analog regimen (Lantus and Humalog), and she has continued counting now that she uses a pump. As a diabetes educator with diabetes herself, Karen Poenisch also is a strong advocate of carb counting and using insulin-to-carb ratios to help correctly judge insulin doses. "Everyone is different," she says. "What works for me may not work for someone else." Learning your individual responses and needs is critical to achieving blood glucose control. Similarly, a pump user himself, Rabbi Meisels advises people to get an insulin pump and to invest the time and effort into getting more and more accurate with carb counting.

It's likely important to not only watch carbohydrate intake but to keep track of fat and protein as well. "I watch my food intake, but I also stay away from fats now because the fat is not good and takes my sugar up," Barbara Baxter, an insulin pump user, states "As I have gotten older, I have found that fat is what affects my blood sugars the most." In all likelihood, using a basal-bolus insulin regimen (achieved with insulin pumps or basal insulins like Lantus plus injections of rapid-acting ones for meals) has made many people more aware of the fact that fats can affect blood sugar levels hours after you eat them, but probably only if you are eating adequate carbs. Fats don't directly get converted into glucose like a portion of protein does, but they can raise your body's resistance to insulin, especially when your carbohydrate intake is higher. This effect usually occurs when the fat is fully digested, often four to six hours after eating. Basal insulin doses seldom have any extra insulin built to cover for the fat hitting your system that late after meals when rapid-acting insulins are mostly out of your system. Using Regular insulin would make the effects of fat less apparent due to its longer duration, but most people have switched to using one of the rapid-acting insulins (e.g., Humalog, NovoLog, or Apidra) instead.

As far as protein goes, it may be converted slowly and ineffectively, but up to about 50 percent of it can eventually be released into your bloodstream as glucose, so it's not uncommon for a large intake of protein to affect blood sugars three to four hours after a meal. Karen Poenisch avoids lots of protein intake at one sitting for another reason. "I don't eat much meat—no more than three ounces per meal," she says. "If I overeat protein, it delays the entry of my carbs, and then my insulin doesn't match well with my carbs."

Coming from an alternate viewpoint, Dick Bernstein believes that keeping your blood sugar levels normal at all times—to keep your glucose excursions the same as nondiabetic friends and family—is the key to being a diabetes survivor. However, he contends that it's almost impossible to avoid spikes in blood glucose if you're eating large amounts of carbohydrates. For his patients, he advocates eating a maximum of six grams of carbohydrate at both breakfast and lunch, with twelve grams allowed for dinner, to follow along with his "laws of small numbers." He says that "small inputs, small mistakes" is the key to winning with diabetes. Taking in a large quantity of carbs at any time, he contends, requires much higher doses of insulin, which are almost impossible to precisely match with the carbs to cover the peaks and the total duration of their glycemic effect. Since his protein intake is therefore a lot higher, he uses Regular insulin for his meals instead.

Gerald Cleveland also limits his carbohydrate intake, but not quite to Dr. Bernstein's extreme. He agrees, however, that the most difficult part is measuring the input of carbs, along with everything else you eat, and getting the insulin dose to match precisely. Another advocate of being careful with your carbs, Anna Maria Gould has experienced that when she eats a large amount of them, her blood glucose goes up, but then it comes down rapidly from the insulin she takes to try to cover it. When she has passed out from a low blood sugar reaction, it has almost always been after a large carb and insulin intake. She says, "I have learned to balance it out better with lower carbs and more protein. The South Beach Diet has taught me this. Rarely do I eat white flour products, rice, macaroni, or pasta. On a lower-carb diet, I also feel more alert and coherent."

If you are an advocate of carb counting, a number of books and other resources are available now to help you learn how to do so more effectively (some of which are listed in the Suggested Reading section at the back of this book). Given that carbs do dictate most of your food-related insulin requirements, if you take the time to learn more about carb counting or at least focus on restricting your intake of them, your reward will be better control of your diabetes.

❧ 21 ❧

Eat Your Cake (but Not Much of It)

An interesting observation arose while Dr. Sheri was interviewing the more than fifty diabetic individuals who are included in this book. For almost all of them who have been living with diabetes since well before blood glucose meters became widely available in the 1980s, desserts consisting of sugary concoctions to this day aren't a routine part of their diets. Most of them had a "no sugar" diet imprinted on their brains from the start of having diabetes, and if they got it early enough in life, they never developed the taste for such desserts. In almost all cases, the old-timers who were brought up with strict diabetic exchanges, no blood glucose meters, and no rapid-acting insulin analogs still eat no (or very few) sugary desserts. For example, Dee Brehm, who has been living with diabetes for 58 years without a single discernible diabetic complication, eats dessert "once every 50 years."

"Insulin is not an instantaneous thing; it takes time to peak. Cake is hard to cover even with rapid-acting insulins," says Al Lewis, a diabetes veteran of almost 70 years. Similarly, after living with diabetes for 63 years, Patricia La France-Wolf also firmly believes that dessert is neither necessary nor easy to manage when it comes to your blood sugars. "It's impossible to figure out how many calories are in pie or how many grams of carbs are in most desserts," she states. "I never eat any sweets," remark both Bob Cleveland and Gladys Dull, the two people living with diabetes the longest of all. Bob adds, "That includes cookies, cake, and all that stuff. Well, I might eat one if I'm really low. Sweets just really don't hold any interest for me. What a lot of people don't realize, though, is that regular carbs can turn into sugar, too. 'Sugar-free' cookies still produce sugar in your blood. You can eat a banana or an apple, and it'll produce sugar. You have to be careful about your diet and the amount of carbs you eat from any source."

Both Bob and Gerald Cleveland eat desserts every once in a while to treat a low blood sugar reaction. What's more, Gerald does eat some ice cream occasionally—usually Edy's sugar-free vanilla ice cream that has reduced fat and calories—because he knows from reading the carton's label that it contains sixteen grams of carbs per half cup, which requires him to take one unit of insulin to cover. Other desserts, though, even ones that are "sugar free," hold little appeal because of their effect on his blood sugars. Recently, he has been trying to educate others in his retirement community about the glycemic effect of desserts (other than ice cream). To prove his point, one day when the usual ice cream was not available, he ate some of the "sugar-free" pie instead, and his blood sugar shot up to 500 even with his usual dose of insulin.

Marcy Shefsky of Newtown, Pennsylvania, who has been living with diabetes 69 of her 74 years, really didn't have a hard time giving up all the candy and other sugary stuff that kids like. "It wasn't hard to say no to it because not eating it was a way of life for me," she states. She was put on a strict "no sugar" diet when her diabetes was diagnosed in 1938. To make up for her restrictions, her father used to go out every Saturday morning to buy her some sugar-free candy. "It was terrible," she recalls, "but I never told him." Nowadays, she is not quite as strict with her diet as she was, but she still doesn't routinely include sugar in it. She provides an occasional birthday cake for one of her grandkids but doesn't indulge in more than a bite of it.

Likewise, Patty Schaeffer advises that if you're young enough to not develop a taste for sweets in abundance, you should keep it that way. There's no doubt that humans usually appreciate sweet-tasting things, likely because carbohydrate intake helps maintain our blood glucose levels and our taste buds recognize the carbs, but how much you eat of such things is more of a habit than anything else. Patty only eats pumpkin pie (which has a relatively low glycemic effect) but hasn't had any lemon meringue pie in the last 40 years. Carolyn Balcom, who was diagnosed in her late 20s, doesn't eat sweet things either, not even many foods with artificial sweeteners in them. "I spent so many years not eating them," she says, "that it has gotten so I don't even like them. My tastes have changed." Jo Allen from Amarillo, Texas, who has had diabetes for 59 of her 75 years, has also never eaten sweets, or even much fat. Carol Sawyer doesn't eat much sugar and never has during her 49 years with diabetes. "My blood sugars are well controlled mostly because of my diet." Blondie Fram doesn't eat anything with added sugar, and for dessert, Grant McArthur and Peter Gariti only eat fruit. After 64 years of diabetes, Jim Arthur's fruit is limited to pears and bananas for the most part. "Oranges have too many carbs," he says. "If I were to eat an orange, I might as well eat some cake because I'd get just as much sugar." He doesn't eat many high sugar foods, though.

Larry Verity, living with diabetes for 31 years, also doesn't usually eat dessert, even though there was a time in his life before he was diagnosed in his early 20s when he expected it. "Now, I don't need or want dessert," he says. "Why eat more calories if you know it's just going to mess up your blood glucose? I don't miss it. I just eat foods I like better, and I'm happy." For herself, Dr. Sheri finds that eating most desserts just isn't worth the extra insulin she has to take or the effort she has to make to stay on top of her blood sugars, and if she ever has any, she prefers to have some fresh fruit anyway (which is what she grew up eating instead of sugary desserts). She indulges in a very occasional piece of ice cream cake (albeit a very small one) on family birthdays, though, which she has found has much less of an impact on her blood sugars than regular cake does.

Only the relative new-timers, along with one or two people with greater diabetes longevity who got diabetes at a much later point in their lives, eat desserts and simply try to cover their glycemic effect with extra rapid-acting insulin. Karen Poenisch admits, "I eat some desserts, but it's hard to figure out how many carbs are in cheese-cake. I have to really want it to eat it. I have figured out how to bolus for chocolate, though: I used a combination bolus on my insulin pump." Others are quite liberal about their intake of foods that most people without diabetes eat, but usually with a caveat. Jim Turner says, "Eat your cake . . . but not much of it."

If you do eat cake or "cheat" on your diet in other ways, act responsibly and try to take enough rapid-acting insulin to cover it without making yourself hypoglycemic. In other words, don't just sit around and feel guilty about what you ate; just take control and treat it as best you can. Patty Schaeffer's advice is to "take an extra injection as needed to cover Christmas dinner." Julie Krupnick, a 28-year diabetes veteran, finds that Krispy Kreme doughnuts are her nemesis. "I have to deal with my cravings to be able to control my blood sugars," she says, also noting that she boluses with her pump to cover any sugary transgression. S. Fasten advises, "If you ever cheat, just correct it and go on.

Everyone I know with diabetes cheats at some point. When I do, I know I'll correct it within three hours." If you don't use insulin, use a blood glucose meter before and several times after any dessert to determine what effect it has on your blood glucose levels. If your sugars go up over 200 mg/dl when you eat it, consider either cutting it out or following Marcy Shefsky's advice: "I take a smidgen of cake—one big forkful is all," she says. Her moderation serves her blood sugars well, as it can also do for you.

🌿 22 🌿

Watch Out for Restaurant Food

Since eating out makes it more challenging to estimate the carbohydrate (as well as protein and fat) content of foods, it's frequently a crap shoot to eat in restaurants. Fast-food restaurant selections typically consist of high-fat, calorie-dense, nutrient-poor choices, along with rapidly absorbed carbohydrate foods, and even meals in sit-down restaurants are typically higher in fat, calories, salt, and sugar than home-cooked versions. The portions at restaurants have also been increasing steadily over the past several decades, with super-sized "value" menus plentiful and inexpensive. If you have any of the usual accompaniments to the main meal at fast-food restaurants, such as French fries, chips, or soda, they can dramatically increase the calories, carbohydrate, fat, and glycemic effect of your meal as well.

Dr. Sheri invariably finds that, for her, eating out at restaurants always requires more insulin to cover it, often for many hours afterward, even when she watches her food intake and makes careful selections. Two major problems with eating restaurant foods are guessing their actual carbohydrate content and dealing with their excessive calorie content, since both factors can affect your blood sugars both immediately after eating and for many hours after you've eaten. By way of example, when at home Dr. Sheri usually eats her vegetables plain or with a little lemon pepper on them, but if you order an equal amount of veggies in a restaurant, it will usually arrive covered with butter or oil, which greatly increases its calorie content. Dr. Steve has a hard time eating out and controlling his blood sugars as well. He says, "I eat too much and usually do not guesstimate the amount of insulin I need very well. Also, the bread basket at the beginning of the meal usually gets me off to a bad start."

The abundance of buffet-style meals, such as all-you-can-eat pizza and unlimited foods at other restaurants, is not at all helpful for people with diabetes either. Chances are you'll end up eating more than you need when you're paying for an unlimited amount of food, and studies have shown that having a wider variety of selections also makes people eat more than they need. Also, you'll likely end up overeating before feeling satisfied if you're loading up on the foods typically found in such restaurants that are high in calories and low in fiber. The lack of vegetables, salad, or fresh fruit not already doctored with extra butter, oil, dressing, or whipped cream only makes your blood sugars harder to control. Not surprisingly, studies have shown that very large meals with high fat and carbohydrate contents result in a major increase in insulin requirements (whether it's insulin that your own body releases or what you give yourself). Dr. Sheri finds it impossible to eat a buffet meal—even one heavy on salads and vegetables—that does not end up negatively impacting her blood sugars for many hours afterward, despite her valiant efforts to keep her blood sugars normal. Dr. Steve says what works better for him, though: "I avoid all-you-can-eat places, and if there is a choice at a buffet place, I order off the à la carte menu even though it's not the best dollar deal." Doing so better controls the size and carb content of your meal.

For Bill King, he finds eating at any sort of social gathering more challenging. "The food is typically laced with fats and sugar," he says. "It takes me combination and extended boluses with my insulin pump to gain control again. You even have to follow up with one-hour and two-hour blood sugar checks and aggressive follow-up after eating out or at a party." He typically finds that if he focuses on the volume of food that he eats—and he tries to limit that—he does best. For example, he remembers one time recently when he went out to eat at an Italian restaurant. "That's what's wrong with this country. I ordered their lasagna," he recalls, "and when the waiter brought it to the table, he told me, 'If you eat the whole thing, it's free.' I was tempted, but I was proud of myself for stopping halfway. Maybe it was fear of gaining another five pounds, combined with my vision of myself as being an athlete that stopped me." Regardless of how he was able to put down his fork, the result was better blood sugar control following his meal!

There are some ways to get around being waylaid by restaurant food, however. Patty Schaeffer has found the secret of what works for her. "We go out for dinner once a week after Saturday Mass, and we've been doing it for at least twenty years. I have records of my blood sugars from 1986 on, and I've tracked my responses to the same restaurants, so I can estimate with fair accuracy how much insulin I need for certain meals." She also tends to eat the same meals over and over, which makes them almost the same as eating at home. Along a similar vein, Gladys Dull eats out at a restaurant once in a while and says, "Most of the time, I can just about guess the effect that a food will have on my sugars." Eating meals out while traveling somewhere new would likely be a completely different story, though, which is why most of the rest of us have more trouble with our blood sugars under those conditions.

❧ 23 ❧

Consider Being a Grazer

Interestingly, if you become a "grazer," or someone who eats small meals and snacks throughout the day, you'll typically end up leaner than someone who eats less often, even if you're eating an equivalent number of calories. Research has shown that eating four to six smaller meals throughout the day may keep your metabolic rate at a higher level, thus increasing your overall energy expenditure for each day, and your risk of developing cardiovascular problems may also be lower. By not becoming too hungry between meals, you will also be less likely to overeat and have problems controlling your blood sugars afterward.

For anyone with diabetes, if you eat only small amounts of food and particularly carbohydrates at any given time, you are more apt to be in the right ballpark when it comes to giving (or releasing) enough insulin to cover what you eat. Jim Turner reports that he eats "lots of small meals" throughout the day that he tries to keep as low carb as possible. He then takes "lots of little shots" to cover his food intake. The only downside of this technique is that short- or rapid-acting insulins can hang around for two to four hours, and you can get overlapping effects of the different doses. If the doses are all small, however, the effect will not be that overwhelming or necessarily cause low blood sugars. For people with type 2 diabetes not on supplemental insulin, small meals and snacks will also likely be beneficial. In all likelihood, with such dietary habits, your pancreas will be able to release enough insulin to cover a little bit of food at a time, rather than being overwhelmed by a lot all at once (particularly carbohydrates).

For insulin users, as long as you don't mind taking extra insulin throughout the day, grazing can work well. For example, like most individuals, Dr. Sheri is most insulin resistant in the morning, but she loves to eat old-fashioned oatmeal with fruit. To do so, she has to take a larger dose of insulin than the number of carbs she eats would normally require at any other time of day, but then once the insulin resistance begins to fade, her sugars start to drop. To deal with this scenario effectively, she takes her insulin and eats breakfast, but then eats again within an hour or two (usually a Nature Valley Trail Mix Bar or a banana) to balance herself out and prevent hypoglycemia. For lunch, she takes everything she plans on eating with her to work, but then she eats it over a two- to three-hour time period, as she has time while she's working. With dinner, she does less grazing, but she makes certain that a large portion of her dinner consists of lower-carb veggies (e.g., broccoli, cauliflower, green beans, and lettuce), and then she doesn't eat again for the rest of the evening. She also tends to check her blood sugars one or two hours after eating and corrects with additional insulin when she goes above 150 mg/dl within an hour afterward.

Although Jessica Ching admits to eating three meals on the weekdays, she also snacks a lot, which really still qualifies as grazing because her meals are not that large. "I take five to eight boluses with my insulin pump most days," she says. "The amounts that I eat vary a lot, and I love being able to eat normally." For her, grazing and having an insulin pump go hand-in-hand, since it's easy for her to give herself extra boluses without having to stick herself yet again. Along the same lines, Dick

Bernstein has had at least one of his patients control her glycemic responses by eating small amounts of protein every two to three hours all day long instead of larger meals.

For people suffering from gastroparesis, eating only small quantities of food will also help keep it moving normally through your stomach and intestines. If you have this diabetes-related complication, large quantities of food result in a sluggish digestive response, one that may make it difficult to cover effectively with insulin injections, without first resulting in hypoglycemia and later having the opposite blood sugar problem. If you eat smaller quantities at any one time, though, you will require less insulin release or a smaller insulin injection, and the margin for error will be much less than when consuming larger amounts of food. Remember that even with grazing, though, if you normally take insulin for the food that you consume, you will still have to take it for small quantities of food as well (albeit smaller doses at any one time).

🎗 24 🎗

Carry a Toothbrush

A secret that we heard from one diabetic survivor, Freddi Fredrickson, who has been living with diabetes for 46 years already, was the recommendation to carry a toothbrush with you at all times. For what purpose, you ask? To brush your teeth after eating to keep yourself from being tempted to eat more, of course. Actually, we're not making fun of this secret, as it's actually a very good suggestion. Lots of things taste bad when you have to mix them in your mouth with the remnants of mint-flavored toothpaste. Dr. Steve recommends having a toothbrush cover as well. "I always keep a toothbrush with a cover in my car and try to brush [without using much or any toothpaste] when I am in light traffic," he admits. "I have to say that it's embarrassing to be seen brushing your teeth in a yellow Porsche, though!"

This secret works well in the evenings, too, after you've finished your dinner. If you go ahead and brush your teeth soon after your meal is done, you should feel somewhat inhibited from eating dessert or snacking some more afterward. "I usually try to brush my teeth within an hour of when we finish dinner," says Dr. Sheri. "That way, I'm a lot less likely to help myself when I'm getting bedtime snacks for my kids or preparing their lunches for school the next day."

There is likely an even more important reason to follow Freddi's advice: People with diabetes are more likely to develop periodontal (gum) disease, and good oral hygiene can help prevent problems. While poor oral hygiene is a factor in gum disease for everyone, having diabetes accelerates the process. Poorly controlled diabetes that contributes to gum disease is one of the leading causes of tooth loss among adults. Circulatory problems linked to diabetes can make your gums more susceptible to infections, which can in turn lead to inflammation of the gums and loss of gum tissue, as well as low-grade infections that can go throughout your body. High glucose levels in saliva also promote the growth of bacteria residing on teeth and gums and plaque formation.

What's more, periodontal problems have actually been linked to a higher incidence of heart disease and strokes. Your risk of heart problems is doubled when you have periodontal disease, unless it's kept under control. The likely link is that oral bacteria can aggregate in the mouth, enter the bloodstream, and then attach to plaque developing in your coronary arteries, thus contributing to arterial plaque formation (not just plaque on your teeth). Periodontal disease also increases a potent clotting agent in the bloodstream called fibrinogen, which increases your chances of getting a blood clot that may cause a heart attack or stroke.

To cut down on plaque formation and excessive bacteria on your teeth (and gums), it is recommended that you brush your teeth at least twice daily and floss between them once a day. However, toothbrush trauma can cause gum recession, so learn how to brush correctly and always use a soft toothbrush. Also, don't smoke, as any type of smoking accelerates the progression of gum disease, as well as heart disease.

PATRICIA LA FRANCE-WOLF, AGE 65, LIVING WITH TYPE 1 DIABETES 63 YEARS

Diagnosed with type 1 diabetes at only 22 months old over 60 years ago, Patricia La France-Wolf decided early on not to let diabetes ruin her life. In fact, her number one secret behind her success is having a good attitude. "I persevere in my life, even when things aren't going good. Nothing stays good all the time, but nothing stays bad all the time either," she remarks. "No matter what happens to you, it will pass." Her outlook is remarkable, particularly given what she has had to live with for over 30 years.

Her kids were only 8 and 10 years old when Patricia went completely blind in 1997. At the time that proliferative diabetic retinopathy caused both of her retinas to detach, she was working as a registered nurse. Since that vocation was no longer an option without her sight, she went back to school and got a master's degree in rehabilitation counseling. Since that time, she has tirelessly worked teaching newly blind people (mostly seniors with macular degeneration, but about a third with diabetes) about how to live well as a blind person, including how to check their blood sugars using talking glucose meters and how to deal with the emotional issues associated with having health problems. She certainly practices what she preaches.

Although she recently retired from the California State Department of Rehabilitation, this Temple City, California, resident still volunteers teaching diabetes education classes for the blind. "I'm out of the house five days a week," she says. "I'm practically as busy as I was before I retired." Another of her longevity secrets is keeping busy, being social, and going out with other people. In fact, she tries to get others to do the same, encouraging newly blind people to enroll in classes at the Braille Institute or local senior centers.

In addition to her positive outlook and desire to educate herself and others about self-care, Patricia also has some other health practices she religiously follows to manage her diabetes. She tells students in her classes that "diabetes can be a DREAM or a nightmare," with "D" standing for "diet," "R" for "responsibility," "E" for "exercise," "A" for "attitude," and "M" for "medicine," all of the aspects of diabetes self-management that she finds best help her manage her own diabetes. "I try to eat only moderate amounts of carbs. I eat most everything I want to eat, but just not large amounts of stuff." She also recommends going to a good diabetes doctor (not an internist) who understands about counting carbs and other important diabetes care techniques. Finally, she feels that she has been blessed with having good medical coverage that has allowed her to choose her own doctors and seek out the kind of medical care that she knew she needed for her diabetes. She sees all of her choices as just part of taking responsibility for her own care, which she thinks is critical to living long and well with diabetes. Given all she has overcome and accomplished in her life, she appears to have better sight than many others with diabetes who fail to see how important taking care of themselves is!

PART FIVE

Exercise Secrets

Exercise Daily
(or Close to It)

Of all the secrets to being successful at living long and well with diabetes, exercise is the one that came up the most consistently as one of the top ones, regardless of how long people had been living with the disease. Given that physical activity can cause low blood sugars—both during and afterward, with a delayed effect—you would think that fewer people would find it important for glycemic control, especially insulin users and people taking certain oral diabetic medications that increase the risk of exercise-related hypoglycemia. However, the majority said that it was one of their primary salvations, particularly before the advent of blood glucose monitors. Dr. Sheri recalls, "I started exercising as a kid way before I ever got a blood glucose meter because it was about the only thing that made me feel better physically. Now, almost 40 years later, it still does! I work out doing various activities at least five to six days a week." Dr. Steve also grew up exercising regularly. He remarks, "Exercise was one of the key things that kept me going."

Bob Cleveland recalls a summer when he was 6 or 7 years old

(over 80 years ago) when his family rented a cabin on a nearby lake. Even then the glucose-lowering effects of exercise were evident to him. "In the two weeks that we were there, I learned how to swim, and I stayed in the water almost all day long. I had been taking lots of insulin, but my mother had to cut back on my doses. She could tell by testing my urine (the only method of monitoring available at the time, albeit an imprecise one). If there was no sugar in it, she cut back on my doses." At least in modern times, we have blood glucose monitors to check actual levels and to make more scientific, calculated dosage changes to compensate.

Even now Bob still experiences the benefits of exercise on his blood sugars. One of the reasons he goes to Florida in the wintertime is so he can be more active. "If I'm at home in Syracuse and the weather is bad, I'd have to take more insulin during the day and my sugars would still run higher. On most days in Florida, I can ride a bike a long way—yesterday I rode twenty miles—and never have to take any rapid-acting insulin. With all that activity, I only needed my basal dose at bedtime." While not everyone gets away with cutting out that much insulin, it certainly highlights the fact that exercise allows your body to take glucose out of the bloodstream without much extra insulin.

Why does exercise help your blood sugars so much? It's because your muscles actually have two separate ways to get glucose into them. When you're resting, insulin works to do it, but during exercise, muscle contractions themselves cause you to take up glucose without the need for insulin (whether you make it yourself or inject it). Thus, exercise always has the potential to lower your blood sugar levels. The only potential downside is that if your insulin levels are too high when you're exercising, your sugars can drop rapidly due to the additive effects of insulin and muscle contractions.

"Exercise makes such a big difference," Rich Humphreys agrees, as does Freddi Fredrickson, who says, "It makes my insulin work much better." Jim Turner also states, "Exercise is key for blood glucose control." At a minimum, Jim plays basketball for a couple of hours at least twice a week ("I'm the oldest guy on the court by ten years," he says), and when he does, he takes much less insulin. The day after, he also eats more carbs for breakfast. Marialice Kern prefers hiking in the California foothills, and she also feels that exercise makes a big difference in her diabetes care. Finally, Gladys Dull says that she knows it makes a difference because before she had a glucose monitor, she only used to get low during her activities—such as cycling, snowmobiling, horseback riding, and more.

Undeniably, engaging in daily (or nearly daily) exercise done consistently makes it easier to manage your blood sugars. Thus, establishing an exercise routine can help you to exercise and balance them more effectively. If you consistently exercise at the same time of day doing a usual activity, by monitoring your sugars before, occasionally during, and afterward, you can establish your glucose response to the activity and determine the best adjustments to make in your food intake and medications. For insulin pump users, disconnecting the pump (or at least lowering basal rates) during activities also helps prevent hypoglycemia because it mimics what a nondiabetic person's body normally does during exercise—when insulin levels go down. For people with type 2, their bodies will be able to lower insulin levels during exercise naturally.

Chuck Eichten believes that he is in better health than most people without diabetes, which he attributes to his regular exercise. Like Dr. Sheri, even before he had a blood glucose meter, he figured out several years into his tenure with diabetes that exercise had a profound effect on his blood sugars. He says, "Exercise has been the biggest savior for me in terms of controlling my blood glucose levels. It functions almost like another insulin dose for me." He admits that even though he doesn't have to exercise regularly nowadays to control his diabetes with an insulin pump, it's still such a habit that he does some type of aerobic exercise—usually cycling or running—for thirty to forty minutes a day. He also tries to make it fairly constant so that his level of activity is about the same because that makes it easier to control his blood sugars.

Although she currently uses Lantus instead of a pump, Dr. Sheri's basal insulin doses are set for her to exercise daily, and she only has to adjust her insulin up on the one or two days a week that she doesn't do any planned activities (other than her normal daily living ones). Her exercise times are not consistent, although any given workout (e.g., an hour of swimming, an hour of cardio machines, resistance training, or stationary cycling) usually varies little from one time to the next, so she already knows each workout's likely effect on her blood sugars, which she can adjust with lower bolus insulin or higher carb intakes (or a combination of both).

For Natalie Saunders, regular morning exercise (usually walking) keeps her blood sugars down for the rest of the day, so she tries to do it consistently. Bernadette McIntyre agrees that she does better with a regular routine at the gym, where she works out at least three to four days a week on the elliptical strider, doing abs, arm and leg resistance work, and run-walking on a treadmill. Larry Verity has developed a similar routine of thirty to fifty minutes of cardiovascular training six days a week, along with some resistance training. He says, "Exercise—you just gotta do it! The Surgeon General's report said that if you can't find time for exercise, you'd better find time for disease." This saying applies to everyone, even people without diabetes.

Conversely, Karen Poenisch states that exercise and its effects on her blood sugars is one of her main struggles with controlling her diabetes. "It affects how my body uses insulin now and over the next two days," she complains. "It affects my basal doses, my insulin-to-carb ratios, everything. I always walk daily on a tread-mill or outside. If I miss doing it or it's not my usual time, it messes everything up." She particularly has trouble doing spontaneous exercise, where she just gets up and does something. "I also need at least twenty minutes before doing any exercise so that I can lower my basal rate on my insulin pump first," she says. Although she firmly believes that daily exercise is important to cut down on the risk of cardiovascular disease, she also advises making it as consistent as possible—that is, same schedule, same amount of exercise—to make blood sugar control easier.

There is no doubt that exercise can also increase the likelihood of experiencing lows both during and after activities—for as long as twenty-four to forty-eight hours afterward. The immediate effect comes from a greater use of blood glucose during exercise, but delayed-onset hypoglycemia often results from greater insulin action in the hours to days following the activity, which is largely attributable to the replacement of glycogen, your muscles' storage form of glucose. Your insulin action will be heightened most in the first couple of hours following an activity and diminish over time as your glycogen is replaced. The most effective way to prevent delayed lows is to make sure that you take in some carbohydrate after the activity, since low-carb diets are known to slow the rate of glycogen repletion. Your body may need very little insulin to take up glucose right after exercise, though, so if you take any, cut back on your usual amount of insulin for the number of carbs you're taking in.

❧ 26 ❧

Live an Active Life

When it comes right down to it, how long you're physically active each day is likely more important than what you do. According to recent studies, participating in close to three hours (170 minutes) of exercise per week at any intensity (i.e., easy, moderate, or hard) improves insulin sensitivity more than if you accumulate only two hours (115 minutes) weekly. The length of your physical activities, therefore, appears to be more important for your blood glucose control than how hard you're working during them.

Thus, to be truly effective, a formal exercise program consisting of thirty minutes a day needs to be combined with more daily spontaneous physical activity, which usually is composed of the activities of daily living like walking. Most of the diabetic individuals who don't engage in any exercise programs per se state that they're very active people in general. Even though a few of the old-timers with diabetes are not especially physically active at present (for health or other reasons), they all feel that being physically active is important to longevity with diabetes and good health, and most have led active lives. By way of example, Mary Sue Rubin does a variety of physical activity. At work, she walks a mile almost every day. She also walks her dogs on weekends, does some gardening, shovels snow (she lives in Maryland), and stretches frequently. "Physical activity is one of my top secrets behind my almost half century with diabetes."

Bob Elder has also been physically active most of his life since before he was an officer in the Marines and diagnosed with diabetes at the age of 23. Long retired and fast approaching 70 years of age and 47 years with diabetes, he states, "I just want to stay active and reasonably healthy and not be dependent on anyone else." With that goal in mind, he plays golf regularly, plays tennis at least once a week, and stays active overall. His cardiologist now has him also doing more aerobic workouts to help lower his blood pressure. Jim Arthur, a regular exerciser until his neuropathy pain has kept him from walking as much in the past four years, says that he has always had active hobbies like golf and basketball. "Now I do water walking and swimming," he says. "It's an easy and good way to exercise. In fact, water walking is especially great when you have neuropathy and loss of balance." Peter Gariti has also always been pretty active. "I like to keep moving," he says. His current activities mainly consist of yard work when the weather permits and mall walking with his wife, although he used to belong to a gym.

Likewise, Carolyn Balcom used to do more regular exercise, but she had been slacking off for various reasons. To make herself more aware of how active she is (or isn't), she has started wearing a pedometer as a reminder to take more steps during the day. For Jane Dohrmann, a pedometer has also become an essential tool for her diabetes management. She says, "Exercise is my biggest hurdle. I *hate* to exercise, and I know it's the one thing I should be doing more of, especially since I am also a heart patient. I have begun to wear my pedometer and do my best to take extra steps to do normal tasks around the house, and we park farther away from stores, et cetera. I need to find a way to do this and keep it up." They both know what they're talking about because studies have shown that women wearing pedometers who have a goal of 10,000 steps per day walk more than others whose only goal was a brisk, thirty-minute walk.

TO PEDOMETER OR NOT TO PEDOMETER— THAT IS THE QUESTION

Probably the best argument for wearing a pedometer is that it has a strong motivational effect. If you have a goal set for each day (such as 10,000 or more steps), and you get near the end of the day and see you only have amassed 5,000, you're more likely to exercise at the end of the day to make up for it. Counting your steps can also be a "social activity." The American Diabetes Association sponsors ClubPed, an online group (www.diabetes.org/ClubPed/index.jsp) that you can join to keep track of your steps, your progress, and your step goals. In addition, a growing, national campaign called "America on the Move" (www.americaonthemove.org) advocates a minimum increase of 2,000 steps per day for everyone and also offers a free online step tracker. Other walking programs can be accessed online, including Web-walking USA (http://walking.about.com/cs/measure/a/web-walkingusa.htm), which allows you to track your virtual progress across the United States on the 5,048-mile American Discovery Trail; AccuSplit, a pedometer manufacturer (www.accustep10000.org); and Step Tracker 2.0 (www.steptracker.com), which allows you to easily share your progress with friends, family, coworkers, and even bloggers, if you so desire.

Before you start, there are a few tips on pedometer use that you should know. For starters, if you clip a pedometer somewhere on the front of your waistband and it does not appear to be accurate, try placing it at the small of your back as some pedometers are less effective if you have extra fat around your waist. Other models can be placed in your pocket (e.g., Omron Healthcare pedometers) or attached around your knee or wrist. Pedometers can vary quite a bit when it comes to overall accuracy and performance. While you may like ones with "bells and whistles" like calorie counters and distance trackers, you're better off with a simpler pedometer that will accurately count the number of steps you take; both calorie counts and distance trackers are often inaccurate.

You can purchase inexpensive pedometers through sporting-goods stores or order them online from various Web sites, including www.americaonthemove.org, www.accusplit.com, www.digiwalker.com, www.walk4life.com, www.steps-to-health.org, and www.pedometer-susa.com. The ones that we would recommend are Omron (HJ-112), Yamax (SW-200 and 701), Sportline (330, 345, and 360 models), New Lifestyles (NL-2000), Walk4Life (LS-2525), AccuSplit Eagle 120XL, and Freestyle Pacer Pro pedometers.

Living with diabetes since childhood, Bernadette McIntyre was raised with physical activity as a part of her upbringing. "My mom was a nurse and my father was a dentist, so they were always interested in health," she recalls. "I remember my mom always said, 'Make sure you exercise,' and my dad said, 'Swim—it's good for you,' whenever we went to the Jersey shore in the summers." In her family, it was all about exercise, exercise, exercise . . . and eat your veggies. "To this day, I still think a key secret to living well with diabetes is to keep yourself active and happy." In addition to her regular workouts at the gym, she also walks the dogs, and she took up golf with her husband about a year ago. "As I age, exercise has become even more a part of my life," she says.

While S. Fasten says that he used to be addicted to working out, now he just does a lot of walking for his job, which helps with his control. Will Speer, Sr., also doesn't do any "scheduled" exercise, but he too has always been very active. "I walk every day, and I always park at the far end of parking lots wherever I go." He says he also hikes regularly with his wife. "I just have an active life," he says. A fellow resident of San Diego with Will (and Dr. Steve), John Rodosevich walks every evening with his wife. "I do upper-body work, too, because it's good for my golf game."

For Paul McGuigan, most of his activity comes from doing projects around the house and yard maintenance. He does golf one or two days a week, though, and other activities occasionally. "I'm into outdoor physical activity, like hiking, nature, and Boy Scout stuff. Golfing is helpful, both psychologically and physically. My wife knows it's what I do, and she doesn't give me grief about golfing on Thursday evenings and Saturday mornings," he says. Matt Besley agrees that it's important to stay active, regardless of how little time you have. "Always do something," he advises. "Exercising really causes your body to react to insulin."

Why is all of this activity such a big part of living long and well with diabetes? Likely, it's because in addition to taking up glucose without insulin being required, any physical activity can make whatever insulin you have circulating in your bloodstream work better for a while afterward, whether it's what your pancreas has released or what you've injected or pumped in. So, your blood sugars will usually stay in better control if you're just active as much as possible, even when you're not formally exercising. Standing up, fidgeting, and taking more steps, all of these activities will use up blood glucose and keep your levels lower.

Blondie Fram admits one of her secrets of living more than 40 years with type 2 diabetes is to keep active. Until her last fall fractured her hip, she had been walking two to three miles in the mall every morning. It bothers her that she has had to slow down some since then, but she still tries to walk as much as possible, just not quite as far. She won't let herself sit back and do nothing, though—which she says is a helpful attitude to have. As a former musician and music teacher, she says, "I still try to get out to concerts and other events as often as I can." Zach Barneis, another individual with type 2, was a serious bike rider until he went over the handlebars and injured his right wrist badly a few years ago. After that, he stopped exercising regularly, although he still realizes its importance. "We bought a treadmill, and I'm getting back into it slowly," he says. "But from experience, I can tell you that it doesn't pay to ever stop. Getting back into it is difficult." Sadly, the latest research shows that fewer than 40 percent of adults with type 2 diabetes, or at highest risk for developing it, who have been advised by their doctors to get more active actually do any regular physical activity at all, even though being active has been proven to be a way to prevent and control the disease.

Moreover, being active can have a positive effect on your mood, stress levels, and self-image, all of which can positively impact your diabetes control when they are improved. Bill King says that being active and seeing yourself as an "athlete" is more about your spirit than your athletic capability. "I'm an athlete," he says, "because when I look in a mirror, I see myself as one. If you have an active lifestyle, you will immediately gain self-esteem." He also runs marathons and trains four to five days a week, so he probably does qualify as a true athlete, but for the rest of you with less ambitious athletic endeavors, you can still benefit from seeing yourself that way. Use your vision of yourself as an athlete to stay motivated to be active every day of your long and healthy life.

❧ 27 ❧

Make It Strenuous

There are certain benefits to be had from doing more intense exercise that some old-timers have recognized. Increasing exercise intensity even briefly works for everyone. For instance, in one study, unfit men and women in their 30s and 40s experienced major gains in their aerobic capacity by doing a total of only six to eight minutes of harder exercise a week. Such results explain the sudden interest in the ROM—The 4-Minute CrossTrainer available in specialized gyms that requires you to work out for only four minutes a day, but at a near-maximal pace. Workouts like those, although strenuous, are not likely to improve your cardiovascular fitness as much as longer sessions of aerobic exercise can, but short, intense work does have its benefits. The same intensity principle applies to almost every kind of exercise you do, from walking to cycling to gardening. In fact, even competitive athletes generally plateau at a certain level of fitness and performance unless they do some version of this heavier "interval" training from time to time.

Dick Bernstein, a 61-year diabetes survivor, says that regular, strenuous exercise is what has kept him looking younger and in better shape than most nondiabetic people his age (73 years old). He exercises every night, but in a nonconventional way. "For resistance training, I do one set with the highest weight I can lift three to four times, and then I use lighter weights to take each set up to twenty repetitions total." For cardiovascular exercise, he says, "If you're in proper cardiac shape, for which you should get tested first, start off easy, but then you should finally get your heart rate above your theoretical max, back off, work it back up, back off . . . as many times as you have time for." He believes that this type of training conditions your heart to work fast, but to slow down to a normal pace quickly (which is, incidentally, a sign of higher levels of cardiovascular fitness). He recommends alternating cardio and upper-body training with lower-body training and other upper-body exercises. "Increasing your muscle mass decreases insulin resistance, which is essential for all type 2s," he explains. "For type 1s, exercise can sometimes complicate diabetes treatment, but is essential for health benefits."

Dr. Sheri, being an exercise physiologist who specializes in diabetes and exercise, has some additional suggestions for gaining the most benefits from your workouts. A research study in the July 2006 issue of *Diabetes Care* tested out the exact type of training regimen she usually recommends. In that study, people with type 2 diabetes already walking over 10,000 steps a day began a program called "Pick Up the Pace," or PUP. It still involved walking, but at increased speeds. Once they measured their usual walking speed (in steps taken per minute measured with a pedometer), they were asked to begin walking for thirty minutes, three times a week, at a pace that was only 10 percent higher than normal (e.g., a usual pace of ninety steps per minute would be upped to about 100 instead). Twelve weeks of PUP training for ninety minutes a week additionally increased their fitness without requiring them to take any extra steps.

Thus, to get the greatest health and diabetes benefits from your aerobic exercise, keep the PUP study in mind. During any activity, you can simply increase the intensity of your exercise for short periods of time (so-called "interval training") to gain more from it. To start with, when you're walking, speed up slightly for a short distance (such as between two light poles or mailboxes) before slowing back down to your original pace. During the course of your walk, continue to include these short, faster intervals occasionally, and as you are able to, lengthen them out to last two to five minutes each (or even up to thirty minutes, like was done in the PUP study). Not only will you become more fit and use up extra calories using this technique, but you also will likely feel more tired when you finish your walk (which is actually a good thing). Over the course of several weeks, you may even find that your general walking speed has increased due to the extra conditioning from your interspersed bouts of faster walking.

Also remember, though, that doing intense exercise may actually cause a rise in your blood glucose levels (which is usually only temporary in type 2s, but that may require some additional insulin to bring down in insulin users). For example, if you have type 2 diabetes and you do ten minutes of strenuous aerobic or resistance training, your blood glucose could possibly rise from a level like 130 mg/dl to 165 or higher. After an hour or two at most, your blood sugars will return to the level where they started, if not lower. It's due to the same release of glucose-raising hormones (like adrenaline) that type 1 diabetic swimmer Gary Hall, Jr., often sees his blood sugars rise from 100 mg/dl to 300 from a twenty-one-second all-out sprint down the length of a fifty-meter (Olympic size) swimming pool during competitions. Since he doesn't make his own insulin, though, he has to inject a couple units of rapid-acting insulin to bring his levels back down to normal. If you do an intense workout, one trick to try to counteract this effect is to do ten to twenty minutes of easier aerobic exercise afterward, which will have a glucose-lowering effect rather than a glucose-raising one.

On the other hand, an interesting recent study showed that if you do a short sprint (e.g., ten seconds) at the end of a moderate aerobic workout, your blood sugars will remain more stable (without dropping) for longer following the activity. The study only followed the first two hours, but likely the effect would be lost shortly after that. Accordingly, Dr. Sheri now frequently advises people who are getting low blood sugar during exercise (but who know that they don't have high levels of insulin in their blood from a recent injection or bolus) to do a short sprint to raise their sugars back into a normal range and prevent hypoglycemia. For her, it works great!

TIPS FOR OPTIMIZING YOUR TRAINING

- Move more all day long to build your overall endurance.
- Intersperse occasional faster intervals into any activity that you do.
- Alternate hard and easy workout days to maximize results and minimize injuries.
- Do at least one longer workout a week to build greater endurance.
- For better glucose control, aim to spend a greater total time being active rather than worrying about your workout intensity.
- If your workouts are short, work out harder during them to use more muscle glycogen.
- Use a full range of motion around your joints during all activities, if possible.
- Cross train by doing a variety of activities, including resistance training, for a greater overall fitness, better motivation, and injury prevention
- Rest at least one day a week (to allow your body to fully repair itself), but avoid taking off more than two days in a row so that your insulin action doesn't decrease too much.

❧ 28 ❧

Erase Your Mistakes with Exercise

Although your muscles account for only about 40 percent of your body weight, they can take up 80 percent of any glucose load that you get through your carb intake. Thus, by enhancing the muscles' capacity to take up glucose with or without insulin, exercise comes closer than anything else to "erasing" your mistakes with your food, insulin, or other medications that lead to hyperglycemia. For example, people can eat more carbohydrate and process it more effectively following hard or prolonged workouts, but usually not at other times.

Much of this effect has to do with improvements in the action of insulin (naturally produced or injected) in your body following physical activity. When your insulin works better, you need less of it to have the same or even a greater glucose-lowering effect. As mentioned, the greatest enhancement in insulin action occurs in the few hours following exercise when your muscle glycogen is most depleted and requires replenishment. During this time, you will likely need considerably less insulin to process any carbohydrates that you eat, and you can get away with eating more carbs after exercise, particularly if it was strenuous and prolonged. In addition, athletic muscles store less excess fat in them, which increases their responsiveness to insulin.

Dr. Sheri finds that her blood sugars react less to her carb intake for several hours or days after physical activity, which is what she would expect. Insulin action actually stays enhanced during most of the time that muscle glycogen is being replaced, which can take as short a time as several hours to replace or as long as two days or more, depending on how much you used. Following long-distance exercise, many people experience greatly enhanced insulin action for at least a day or two, although the effect diminishes over time. Eating carbs during this period of time is likely to have less than the usual impact on your blood sugars.

As discussed earlier in this book, Bob Cleveland finds he can go all day on his long-acting Lantus insulin only when he's cycling. Many other diabetic athletes over the years have told Dr. Sheri similar things. Very few of them use much short- or rapid-acting insulin when they're physically active over an extended period of time because of the muscles' ability to take up glucose without insulin during exercise. Then they have to watch out for lows that hit them after the exercise is over, during the time when their bodies are replacing muscle glycogen.

"Exercise is the biggest thing to do," says Jim Turner. "It will erase so many mistakes." His insulin requirements are much lower during and for at least a day after a good workout. "And I eat more carbs, too," he says. Similarly, Bill King's strategy is to start with good blood sugar control and earn the right to eat something like a dessert—by working out first. "I still limit the quantity I eat, though," he says.

Many others, both type 1s and type 2s, who use insulin are able to cut back on their doses depending on their amount of activity. As Chuck Eichten has found, exercise can often substitute for another insulin dose, and for anyone who doesn't have to take insulin, it can make naturally produced insulin work so much better that the effect is similarly positive for type 2s. Robert Mandell, who has only been using insulin to control his type 2 diabetes for the past six or seven years, says, "If I can get in a week of regular exercise, at night I don't need any insulin even though I normally take ten units of NPH then."

If your blood sugars are running consistently above normal any given day, you can often get them back into a more normal range with some exercise. Many regular exercisers with diabetes (and who take insulin) know that if their blood sugars are over 300 mg/dl, they can give a unit or two of rapid-acting insulin and exercise, and the glucose-lowering effect of exercise will be all the more enhanced. "In the past, I have been near 400, taken half the rapid-acting insulin I normally would, gone out to exercise for forty-five minutes, and been near 100 when I was done," says Dr. Sheri. You have to be careful, though; always take much less insulin than you'd normally need to bring you back down to normal. These days, her blood sugars seldom exceed 250 mg/dl, but she keeps the practice in mind. "Oftentimes if I'm around 150 at bedtime and want to be closer to 100, I can choose to either take a unit of Humalog or ride my stationary cycle at an easy pace for twenty to thirty minutes. I usually choose the latter, and it works really well—usually twice as fast as the insulin ever does." If you do a moderately paced exercise, even ten minutes may be enough to lower glucose levels, but avoid really intense workouts that may temporarily raise glucose levels when you're trying to lower them instead.

Endorphins, another natural "eraser" of glycemic mistakes, are mood-enhancing hormones that bind to your brain's natural receptors and cause feelings of euphoria or a "second wind" after you have been exercising for a while. There is evidence that endorphins may actually improve your body's insulin action, thereby reversing or decreasing insulin resistance as well. In fact, endorphin release may be a major mechanism in the enhanced insulin sensitivity attributable to moderate exercise training. If that's the case, go for maximal endorphins on a daily basis to control your blood sugars, and as a side benefit, you will be less depressed and anxious and enjoy a greatly improved mood.

Finally, even though physical activity will allow you to be a little more slack in your diet and still control your blood sugars, this effect works only up to a point. Diabetes is not just a carbohydrate-processing disorder; it is also a disorder of blood fats, which when elevated can contribute to the development of plaque formation in arteries and circulatory problems throughout your body. Your food intake can affect your glucose levels *and* your blood fats, as can your exercise habits, so optimize them by balancing your exercise and your diet for the greatest longevity.

❧ 29 ❧

Compete with Yourself

U ntil a recent back injury forced him out of the water for a while, Al Lewis was a competitive master's swimmer, and athletics have played a major role in doing well with diabetes for 69 years. Even at the age of 73, he feels it's important to be very competitive with yourself. "I'm even more competitive with diabetes than I am with other swimmers," he says. "It's all about being successful with diabetes." For him, exercise has been a big part of his success; in fact, he lists "exercise" as the number one secret of his longevity with diabetes. "If you're successful in controlling your diabetes, it engenders a drive to be in better control," he admits. Another avid exerciser, Chuck Eichten, also agrees that wanting to succeed or excel with diabetes is good, but that it can potentially be dangerous as well. "I found myself taking it to the nth degree. If a 60 blood sugar is good, why wouldn't a 58 be better?"

Although Dr. Sheri is purely a recreational athlete at this point in her life, she has to agree with Al's competitive edge—she also ranks exercise first on her list of her longevity secrets—but admits that you have to be moderate about it like Chuck has discovered. She remarks, "People with diabetes certainly have a higher risk of getting orthopedic injuries—any type of inflammation of joints and tendons—so you can't go overboard with competing with yourself and others if you want to keep exercising over the long haul." The better her control has become over the years, though, the greater her desire to keep it that way or better, although she moderates herself in this regard. "I'm always looking for more information about better ways to keep diabetes in check," she says. "For those of us with goal-oriented personalities and diabetes, we often use athletics to push ourselves harder. My primary goal at this point, though, is just to be able to keep exercising almost daily, which means that I can't push myself so hard that I get an overuse injury that sidelines me."

Al, Chuck, and Dr. Sheri are not the only diabetic athletes with the desire to reach loftier goals, even if they aren't necessarily old-timers. For instance, Gary Hall, Jr., developed type 1 diabetes in 1999 at the age of 24 between his first and second Olympic games, and yet he went on to train for and win a gold medal in fifty-meter freestyle swimming (and other team events) in the 2000 and 2004 Olympic Games, even after his first diabetes physician told him his swimming career was over when he was diagnosed. Instead of giving up, Gary found himself a diabetologist with a more modern outlook on sports participation, Dr. Anne Peters, and he has yet to let diabetes slow him down. At age 29, he became the oldest U.S. male in eighty years to win gold when he defended his fifty-meter freestyle title at the 2004 Olympic Games. He is currently training for the 2008 Olympics, which will be his fourth one, his third since his diabetes diagnosis. Similarly, Sir Steven Redgrave, a five-time Olympic gold medalist in rowing for Great Britain, was diagnosed with diabetes after his fourth Olympic victory, yet he pushed himself and learned how to manage his diabetes effectively enough to win a fifth gold in the 2004 Sydney Olympic Games.

Other elite diabetic athletes like Kris Freeman, a cross-country skier, competed in the 2006 Winter Olympic Games despite the rigors of long-distance endurance training. When his diabetes was diagnosed in 2000 during the height of his competitive season, his doctor also told him that his skiing career was over, but he defiantly strapped his skis back on the same day and went out to train. In many ways, having diabetes has simply made Kris a more regimented and determined athlete, one who is dedicated to living as healthy a lifestyle as possible. Moreover, many athletes with diabetes (both past and present) have successfully participated in professional and elite sports, including Jay Leeuwenburg and Jonathan Hayes (football), Chris Dudley (basketball), Adam Morrison (basketball), Chris Jarvis (rowing), Jason Johnson (baseball), Missy Foy (ultra-distance runner), Zippora Karz (ballet), Michelle McGann (golf), Bill Talbert (tennis), Jay Handy (Ironman triathlons), and Per Zetterberg (soccer), just to name a few of the very many.

A nurse with diabetes since 1972, Paula Harper started the International Diabetic Athletes Association (IDAA), which later changed its name to the Diabetes Exercise & Sports Association (DESA, found at www.diabetes-exercise.org) so that it includes both insulin users and others with diabetes or prediabetes who aren't insulin-requiring. When she founded it in 1985 out of her own home, she was heavily involved in distance running and cycling, but she found it difficult to find any solid information on how to integrate exercise into her diabetes management. Before glucose monitoring became widespread around that time, most physicians recommended that individuals with diabetes not participate in endurance events such as marathons or 100-mile bike races. Following Paula's fifth successful marathon race in 1980, she had "I run on insulin" printed on the back of a T-shirt, and she soon found others doing the same thing, which finally led her to found this organization to bring together diabetic exercisers at all levels of competitiveness. To this day, DESA continues to give athletic achievement awards annually to diabetic exercisers with the greatest accomplishments, who can serve as inspirations to all individuals with any type of diabetes.

Another marathoner, Bill King, had a father who was an American marathon champion. Bill himself had run three marathons prior to developing diabetes, and he planned to keep running after his diagnosis. Adjusting to doing the training mileage needed for effective marathoning with diabetes took some time, but once he got the hang of it, there was no stopping him. "I went on an insulin pump, and for the first time I was able to finish my run without having to stop at Wawa [food market] for something to treat my lows," he recalls. "I ran a half marathon and then the Philly marathon 12 years after getting diabetes. I ran a 3:12 on my first marathon with diabetes. It was just so amazing to be able to get back into the groove of running." He has done more than that, now having run seventeen marathons on insulin. After he qualified for his first Boston Marathon and figured out a way to glue a blood glucose meter onto a wristband so that he could check his blood sugar without stopping and without relying on someone else to meet him at a water stop with a meter. He admits that during that event, his insulin levels were too high, and he experienced a significant low at mile 17 (out of 26.2 miles total). "I needed a better plan," he says. He continued to work with his basal rates on his pump and was able to perfectly balance his sugars during the next year's event.

Finally, others have even more extreme athletic goals. Dave Nevins, now a resident of Stika, Alaska, who has been living with diabetes for 31 of his 43 years, recently undertook a Utah border-to-border ride that covered 465 miles of challenging terrain to raise awareness about diabetes. In 2007, Tom Seabourne was the

RUN A MARATHON? ARE YOU CRAZY?

Given the burgeoning interest that the public at large appears to have with running that infamous 26.2 endurance race, it's likely that other individuals with type 1 and type 2 diabetes will "hear the call" and decide to train for one. That's exactly what happened to Arkansas former governor Mike Huckabee after he was diagnosed with type 2 diabetes a few years ago. More races than ever before are put on as fundraising events, and although elite runners take the prizes home, many other individuals are winning by simply participating. Marathons times for the middle-of-the pack runners have been slowing down for a couple of decades now, and the average time for completing one (as of 2005) was 4:32 for men and 5:06 for women, including more than 384,000 finishers from around 314 marathons around the country.

You can't run a marathon without first doing a copious amount of run training, which likely will not be appropriate for everyone with diabetes (particularly foot nerve damage). However, if you're willing and able to take the challenge, we'd like to send you off to train with a little more knowledge about training properly and preventing overuse injuries. Accordingly, before you start, please research training schedules with appropriate mileage buildup and other strategies by talking to other marathoners or visiting online resources like the following:

www.marathontraining.com/marathon.html
www.bostonmarathon.org/BostonMarathon/MarathonTraining.asp
www.nycmarathon.org/training/trainingschedule.php
www.runnersworld.ltd.uk/marathon.htm
www.jeffgalloway.com/training/marathon.html
www.halhigdon.com/marathon/Mar00index.htm

We'd like to add that balancing your diabetes effectively with training as strenuous and prolonged as marathon training is an individual thing—no one strategy works best for everyone. If you'd like more information about participating in run or marathon training as an insulin user, please consult Dr. Sheri's first book, *The Diabetic Athlete*. For additional advice, connect with other diabetic runners through the Diabetes Exercise & Sports Association (www.diabetes-exercise.org; [800] 898-4322; desa@diabetes-exercise.org) or the Diabetes Sports & Wellness Foundation (www.dswf.org; Jay Handy, triathlete, president at [608] 334-1350 or jay@dswf.org).

first person with type 1 diabetes (diagnosed in his 40s, but first misdiagnosed with type 2) to compete in the grueling cycling event, Race Across America, in the solo division, but Team Type 1 has competed in this race and won the corporate division the past two years running. Founded and headed by Phil Southerland of Atlanta, Georgia, who has lived with diabetes for all but the first 7 months of his 25 years, Team Type 1 includes eight diabetic cyclists taking turns sprinting on a cycle twenty-four hours a day for almost six days to cover the more than 3,000 miles from Oceanside, California, to Atlantic City, New Jersey. To put it in perspective for you non-cyclists, this race is twice the distance of the Tour de France, but riders complete it in far less time. Their goal is to demonstrate that diabetes is an inconvenience, but exercise is the best way to manage your blood glucose.

Another extreme adventurer, Will Cross, who has been living with diabetes since the age of ten, accomplished his primo goal in May of 2006 when he became the first person with type 1 diabetes to reach the top of Mount Everest, the tallest mountain in the world, on his third attempt. This achievement was the culminating adventure of his plan to crest the summits of the seven tallest mountains of the world, along with trekking across both the South and the North Poles. While not all of us with diabetes are quite that extreme, the need to conquer mountains can be considered analogous to our extreme desire to control and conquer our diabetes.

❧ 30 ❧

Maintain Your Weight

Excess body weight is associated with a greater risk of many health problems, and even though it may not be the direct cause of all of them, losing body fat or maintaining your body weight are considered important goals, and exercise plays an important role in reaching these goals. For example, regular physical activity can prevent you from developing type 2 diabetes in the first place or reverse prediabetes, even if you're at higher risk for either health condition. Moreover, weight loss can also help control diabetes in many individuals, regardless of what type of diabetes they have. In a recent reanalysis of the Diabetes Prevention Program (designed to prevent type 2) published in *Diabetes Care* in the fall of 2006, weight loss was most directly correlated to a decreased risk of developing the disease. Likely more importantly, weight loss was predicted by how much exercise people did, and only the ones who continued to exercise after the trial ended were able to maintain their new, lower body weights. Although exercise can't prevent type 1 diabetes, it can prevent a condition dubbed "double diabetes" by reversing or preventing an insulin-resistant state (more common to type 2) in sedentary individuals with type 1, making it easier for them to effectively control their diabetes and prevent acute and long-term health complications.

When it really comes down to it, where you store excess body fat is more important than how much you have. Visceral fat stored deep within your abdomen (the proverbial "beer belly") is the worst type of body fat with regard to diabetes control because it makes your insulin work less effectively. Luckily, both moderate aerobic exercise and resistance training (done even only twice a week) can result in losses of visceral fat that dieting alone doesn't cause. What's more, you can be fit regardless of your body weight and gain almost all of the associated health benefits of having a higher fitness level without struggling to lose weight and keep it off simply by choosing to be regularly physically active.

Keeping your weight down is not the only cure for decreased insulin action (you can be thin and insulin resistant or fat and have good insulin action), but the behaviors that help you keep your weight in a more normal range (like regular exercise) are likely what are going to benefit your diabetes control the most. For Zach Barneis, going on a strict diet after his type 2 diabetes diagnosis and losing about thirty-five pounds in six months kept him off of insulin for a long while, and exercise played an important part in his being able to lose the extra weight. Likewise, Robert Mandell says, "When I was diagnosed with type 2, my doctor told me to lose weight. I actually controlled my diabetes for about the first 15 years with diet and exercise alone, and I lost twenty pounds. I was walking and jogging five days a week and covering about five miles a day."

Dick Bernstein contends that your body fat will not break down in the presence of a substantial level of insulin. Insulin responses can vary greatly from person to person (or none at all is produced in type 1 individuals), but more refined carbohydrate foods (which are low in dietary fiber) evoke a stronger and/or more rapid insulin reaction. Consumption of natural fiber with carbohydrates can reduce the extreme blood sugar reactions described above. Low-fat diets cause quicker digestion and absorption of carbohydrates in the form of sugar. By adding some fats to the diet, digestion and absorption is slower, and the insulin reaction is moderated. Perhaps a third to a half or more of our population is unable to process carbohydrates—sugars and starches—effectively. In many people it's due to genetics, with lifestyle contributing to the condition. This can be termed insulin resistance, or IR. Like many problems, IR is an individual one, affecting different people different ways. You must determine if you are carbohydrate intolerant, and if so, to what degree. Blood tests will only diagnose the problem in the later stages, but the symptoms may have begun years earlier.

As we now know, insulin has many functions. While it can't get glucose into the muscle cells efficiently when muscle becomes insulin resistant, insulin still performs its other tasks, including converting carbohydrates to fat and storing them in fat cells, along with inhibiting stored fat from being released and used as a fuel for the body. In a normal person, as much as 40 percent of the carbohydrates eaten may be converted to fat, depending on your calorie intake. If you're insulin resistant, that number may be much higher. As a result, when you have to take higher insulin doses or your body has to release more to cover food intake, it's much more likely that you'll store extra body fat as a result.

So, if you desire to lose weight, eating few carbs that require either greater release or doses of insulin will make it easier to lose weight. "A low-carb diet, in addition to lowering your blood lipids and your blood glucose, will also help you stay thin," Dick Bernstein confirms. Other individuals have also noticed that they start gaining weight if they take too much insulin. "I do limit my carbs because then I find that I can take less insulin and don't gain weight," says Barbara Baxter, while Jo Allen attributes her weight staying down all of her adult life to the fact that she doesn't eat desserts (which would indeed require higher doses of insulin). Marc Blatstein also realizes that he's been gaining too much weight for good health. "I have gone through periods where I didn't watch the portions," he admits, "and I gained weight. In the past six years, I've gained thirty pounds, but now I am aggressively working to shed this extra baggage by watching my portion control." Larry Verity, too, experiences changes in his weight with higher insulin doses, so he tries to keep his daily insulin as low as possible to prevent excess weight gain. Experiencing frequent hypoglycemia that has to be treated can also cause you to gain weight, so preventing excessive lows is better for this reason alone (not to mention all the other ones).

Dan Spinazzola also says that vanity helps with his weight management. He has a thirty-eight-inch rule. "If my pants get tight," he says, "I refuse to buy a pair with a thirty-nine- or forty-inch waist." In the past year, he has lost about twelve pounds total, which he attributes to a combination of using Byetta and having a positive mental attitude. Dr. Sheri has a similar rule about her clothing. "I refuse to buy a larger size of anything." To this day, she still fits in the same clothes that she wore at the end of high school and throughout her college years, and her weight has remained stable—plus or minus five pounds—the entire time. Even during each of her three pregnancies, she exercised throughout and watched her food intake so that she was back to her normal weight within eight weeks following each one. Many other long-timers with diabetes, like Gladys Dull, Dee Brehm, and Jo Allen, have retained their svelte figures throughout their lives, largely due to their diligence in controlling diabetes with diet and exercise. "I know I'd be a lot heavier if I didn't have diabetes," agrees Natalie Saunders. Thus, having diabetes just gives you another good reason to watch your weight and prevent the common, but not inevitable, middle-age spread.

RICHARD "DICK" BERNSTEIN, AGE 73, LIVING WITH TYPE 1 DIABETES FOR 61 YEARS

There are few diabetes professionals as dedicated to educating people about living well with diabetes as Dick Bernstein, MD, a resident of Mamaroneck, New York. His desire to help others living with the disease stems from his own experiences in helping himself to overcome the ravages of diabetes. His diabetes was mishandled by his doctor from the start, as he was put on an American Diabetes Association (ADA)-backed high-carb, low-fat diet, which required that he take huge doses of insulin, kept him on a blood sugar roller coaster, and sent his triglycerides (blood fats) sky-high.

By 1969, after having had diabetes for over 20 years and in what should have been the prime of his life, Dick was experiencing so many diabetic complications that he appeared chronically ill and prematurely aged—basically, he felt like an old man. His eyes, kidneys, heart, nerves, and joints were all being severely impacted, and given the large amount of protein already showing up in his urine, his life expectancy was likely less than five years.

"I was the victim of the American Diabetes Association's guidelines and procedures," he says. He pointed out all the health problems he was having to his diabetologist, who was then president of the ADA, but he was inevitably told, "Don't worry; it has nothing to do with your diabetes. You're doing fine." His quality of life was suffering, and realizing that his life would be over soon if he didn't take action (and he had three small children he wanted to see grow up), Dick started working out at a local gym at his father's suggestion, but found he couldn't gain any muscle mass. Finally, in 1969, he came upon an ad in *Lab World* for a machine that measured glucose levels in blood, but that was only available to physicians. His wife was one, but he was still an engineer at that point, so he had to order one for himself under her name.

With the help of this early (and very large) blood glucose-monitoring device, Dick was finally able to confirm through testing about five times a day that his blood sugars were routinely swinging between highs of over

400 mg/dl and lows of 40. Through trial and error, he learned that carbs affected his blood sugars more than anything else, so he started cutting back on them. Over the next couple of years, he felt and looked better, but his complications remained. Desperate for a way to reverse them, he searched exercise studies done on animals, hoping that being active would lower or reverse complications. "What I found instead," he recalls, "is that many studies in animals showed that if you lower their blood glucose, you can reverse complications." He put himself onto a low-carb, high-protein diet, combined with basal/bolus insulin dosing. After a few years of optimal blood glucose control, his blood fats were improved and the protein in his urine was back to normal.

After sharing his remarkable results with his doctor, Dick asked what the physician would do for his other patients. He replied, "First of all, I can't have them measuring their own blood glucose (instead of coming in once a month), and I wouldn't be able to get them to inject insulin five times a day, since they don't want to do it once a day now." After encountering such resistance, the young engineer tried submitting his remarkable findings to many different research journals, only to be repeatedly rejected and ridiculed. He also tried to get the word out about the importance of blood sugar control through other avenues, like joining some of the ADA's lay committees, but the whole organization was apparently opposed to blood glucose monitoring at home (at that time).

In 1977, Dick decided to give up his engineering job and become a physician. "I couldn't beat 'em, so I had to join 'em," he remarks in his book, *Dr. Bernstein's Diabetes Solution* (3rd Edition). "With an "MD" after my name, my writings might be published, and I could pass on what I had learned about controlling blood sugar." In 1983, he finally opened his own medical practice, and since that time he has helped thousands of people with diabetes live healthier lives. Remarkably, he was right on the money about the importance of optimal blood glucose control (and we're all thankful to have his advice and home blood glucose monitoring to help us keep it that way). His goal is to have no more spikes in blood glucose than a non-diabetic person. As he says, "That's what it takes to be a survivor."

PART SIX

Medication and Technology Secrets

31

Always Take Your Medications

Regardless of which type you have, diabetes results in a progressive loss of beta cells and a lessening of your insulin-producing capacity over time, if your blood sugars are not within normal levels at all times. All people with type 1 diabetes (even slower-onset adults with type 1) and at least 40 percent of people with type 2 must give themselves insulin (be it injected, pumped, or now inhaled) to control their blood glucose levels. If your blood sugar is quite high when you are diagnosed (greater than 250 mg/dl) with type 2 diabetes, your physician may choose to start you on insulin immediately, although the doses may later be decreased or withdrawn if your lifestyle changes by themselves are effective at controlling your diabetes. Starting on insulin immediately can allow you to rapidly achieve good control and may have a positive residual effect: When people with type 2 diabetes are started on insulin early, they are not likely to still need supplemental insulin a year later (although at some later date, they may need it again). In addition, being put on insulin for type 2 diabetes is not a sign that you have somehow personally failed.

If you are taking insulin, it's important that you don't skip it. Both Dr. Sheri and Dr. Steve admit that they probably stayed out of diabetic ketoacidosis (caused by greatly elevated glucose levels and ketone formation due to insulin deficiency, more common in type 1s) while growing up with diabetes without the benefit of glucose monitoring only because, no matter what, they always took their insulin injections. Many other long-time survivors say the same thing, including Gladys Dull, who in the past 83 years has never missed a shot. The same goes for Marcy Shefsky, living with diabetes for more than 69 years, who admits, "I never fail to take my insulin shot." Vena Petrotta has been taking insulin only a decade less long (but always regularly), and both she and Bernadette McIntyre emphatically say, "I'd never skip my shots!" Freddi Fredrickson says she has always taken her insulin, even when it was just one shot a day in the early years, and Barbara Baxter advises people to "always take your insulin" as one of her longevity secrets.

Obviously, taking your insulin injections (if you require them) is a key secret of success. For all of these individuals, even if their doses weren't always right, the mere fact that they did have some insulin on board at all times helped prevent some acute problems with their blood sugars and likely some of the longer-term ones as well. Many of the longest-living people with diabetes have heard stories about others failing to take their insulin, and most of them react with disbelief. "I have heard of some kids who got into their teens and started skipping their insulin," says Jim Arthur, by way of example. "I'm amazed that they'd go several days without insulin. Never in 64 years of having diabetes have I ever missed an insulin shot."

On the other hand, taking a dose that close to what you actually need is important as well. By way of example, Dr. Steve tells of an insulin dosing fiasco that happened to him after his diabetes diagnosis in 1970. "After I was moved out of the ICU into a regular hospital room, a new nurse gave my injection," he recalls. "She came in with what looked like a huge horse syringe that looked like a large pump squirter that I used for water fights with the kids on my block. The injection really hurt because of the large volume of insulin that was forced into my thigh. A short time later, the doctor assigned to take care of me (who wasn't a diabetes specialist) came in my room. I asked him why the shot was so large, but he was puzzled." To make a long story short, the nurse had misread the doctor's order, and instead of giving the teenage Dr. Steve 15 units of insulin (hand-written very sloppily as "15U"), she had given him ten times that much, or 150 units. When they realized her mistake, all hell broke loose. "They put me back in the ICU, stuck some more IVs in me, made me drink very sweet fluids, and tested my blood sugar every five or ten minutes for several hours." To avoid similar errors, most hospitals now have a rule that the word "units" must be written out completely and not indicated by just a capital "U."

There is no doubt that insulin itself has changed dramatically since its discovery in 1921. It wasn't until 1936 that longer-acting insulins (e.g., protamine zinc, or PZI) were available at all, and before that time, people often had to wake up during the night to inject themselves with short-acting insulin. All of the earlier insulins were derived from animal sources (beef and/or pork, mostly), and human synthetic insulins made entirely in a laboratory from human DNA were not available until 1983. The switch to these newer insulins has allowed people to avoid having as many serious or allergic reactions like many experienced with the beef/pork varieties.

There are so many more kinds of insulin available now that you would really be remiss not to at least attempt to gain better control over your blood glucose levels by using the different insulins to your advantage. You can learn to use different ones strategically, depending on what you're eating or doing on a particular day. For instance, Regular insulin used to be the only one available to cover meals and snacks, but its onset and peak are too slow to cover most carbohydrate loads. So, if you're eating more rapidly absorbed carbs, you can benefit from using a rapid-acting insulin analog instead to better match your insulin with your blood glucose peaks.

Three rapid-acting insulin analogs (all synthesized and slightly altered forms of human insulin) are now on the market: Humalog (the first one approved by the FDA in 1997), NovoLog, and, most recently, Apidra. In addition, intermediate-action insulins like NPH (Humulin N) can be used to cover both basal needs and some meals (like lunch), but have become less popular than basal-bolus regimens that better mimic the normal release of insulin from the pancreas. Truly basal insulins, though, are not intended to cover much beyond your non-food-related insulin needs and are nearly peakless; the widely used ones today are Lantus and Levemir. The usual time to onset, peak, and total duration of the various insulins are compared in the table that follows. Keep in mind that for all injected insulins, smaller doses are generally absorbed from your skin and available in your bloodstream more rapidly than large doses.

COMPARING THE ACTION OF INSULIN AND INSULIN ANALOGS

Insulin	Onset	Peak	Duration
Humalog/Novo Log/Apidra	10–30 minutes	0.5–1.5 hours	3–5 hours
Regular (R)	30–60 minutes	2–5 hours	5–8 hours
Exubera (Inhaled)	10–30 minutes	0.5–1.5 hours	5–8 hours
NPH (N)	1–2 hours	2–12 hours	14–24 hours
Lantus	1.5 hours	None	20–24 hours
Levemir	1 3 hours	8–10 hours	Up to 24 hours

With the rapid-acting insulin analogs, your dose can be given after meals—when you presumably know precisely how many carbs you have eaten—just to cover the food you actually ate. Dr. Steve says, "I usually give my fast-acting insulin towards the end of my meals, unless I'm high beforehand." If your meal is lower in carbs or just contains more slowly absorbed ones (like legumes), or if you take Symlin, taking your insulin sooner can result in hypoglycemia before enough of the food is digested. Rapid-acting insulins make correction of elevated blood sugars a lot quicker than it used to be with just Regular. Most insulin users take corrective doses to bring down glucose levels between meals as well. Grant McArthur acknowledges getting more lows when he used Regular than he does now with NovoLog used on a sliding scale, likely because of the newer insulin's shorter duration.

Dick Bernstein usually uses the older Regular insulin, however, and he advises his patients following his low-carb diet to do so as well. Protein affects your blood glucose, but its effect is just not as immediate as with carbs, since protein takes longer to digest, which is why Regular insulin probably works better for that diet. Also, less than 50 percent of the protein ultimately gets converted into glucose. Dick does use Humalog to correct any blood glucose elevations, and then he injects it straight into his muscle to speed its rate of absorption. In general, he finds its absorption to be less predictable than Regular insulin, though, along with being 50 percent more potent. "You should never use Humalog if you have gastroparesis (delayed stomach emptying)," he advises, "because it will likely cause hypoglycemia before your food is absorbed." He also finds NovoLog to be slower in action than Humalog, but faster than Regular, so he really finds no place for it in his regimen.

In addition, the first inhaled insulin, Exubera, was approved by the FDA in 2006 and mimics the usual action of rapid-acting insulin analogs, although its onset may be slightly more rapid than the analogs and its duration more similar to Regular. Exubera is designed for people with type 1 and type 2 diabetes to take just before meals. In type 1s, longer-acting insulins are still required to cover basal insulin needs, though. One problem with using inhaled insulin is that the dosing is less precise, and for tightly controlled people on insulin, its use may complicate their glycemic control. Other inhaled insulins, such as MannKind Corporation's new Supra-Rapid Acting Insulin delivered by their Technosphere System, are currently in development, as are other alternative forms of insulin including mouth sprays and insulin patches.

Other people have benefited from the smoother actions of the new long-acting basal insulins that have only been available since 2001. Ultralente, which lasted up to forty-eight hours or more, has been replaced by Lantus and Levemir, both lasting no more than twenty-four hours in most individuals. "I don't have bad lows anymore now that I'm on Lantus," Rich Humphreys reports. Although Bob Cleveland only takes one bedtime dose of nineteen units and Dee Brehm only takes ten units then, many other long-living people using either of these insulins take a dose twice daily even though Lantus calls for once-a-day dosing. When you're taking small doses of insulin, Lantus may not last the promised twenty-four hours, although it generally does in people who take much larger doses. You may consider taking twice daily doses of Lantus if you find that it doesn't last a full day for you. Your AM and PM doses don't necessarily have to be evenly split. For instance, Gerald Cleveland takes ten to twelve units at bedtime, but only three units in the morning, while Dr. Sheri takes six units at night and ten in the A.M., and Natalie Saunders gives herself eight and six units at those times, respectively.

As an alternate regimen, insulin pumps provide a constant, preset basal amount of insulin, with boluses given for food intake. The insulin used in pumps is usually a rapid-acting insulin analog or still occasionally Regular or other insulins (e.g., a mix of Regular and Humalog in one person's case). Pump use requires vigilance over your diet and more frequent blood glucose monitoring (to catch problems early), but many people feel that using one has improved their quality of life. For instance, Carol Sessions says she no longer experiences "crashing lows" now that she uses an insulin pump, which makes her overall control much better.

No matter what your insulin regimen, taking insulin nowadays is so much easier than it used to be. The old-timers like the Cleveland brothers, Dick Bernstein, Al Lewis, Jim Arthur, Dee Brehm, and others tell stories about having to sharpen their needles on a whetstone and having to boil their glass syringes after each use. "In 1949, the syringes cost $5 each, which was lots for those days, so you used one forever," remembers Dee Brehm. "The needles were prone to getting barbs when you sharpened them, though," says Jim Arthur, "and that's tough on a 10-year-old" (his age at diagnosis). Carol Sessions remembers using cream of tartar to make her syringe's plunger slide better by sprinkling it in the top, and Peter Gariti recalls having to store his glass syringes in an old peanut butter jar filled with rubbing alcohol with cotton at the bottom of it. Although Dr. Sheri, Dr. Steve, and many others remember practicing giving oranges injections in the hospital to learn how to give shots, as well as the glass syringe boiling routine, the two of them were lucky enough to get diabetes late enough to avoid the mega-needles that were so big that, by comparison, one of today's needles would likely fit completely inside of the original versions.

Even though Larry Verity remembers having a fear of shots because they were more like giving intramuscular injections (instead of just going into the fatty layer below the surface of the skin), and he thought that they hurt a lot, not everyone felt that way. Even after 64 years' worth of shots, Jim Arthur says, "You imagine injections to be worse than they are. Taking insulin is not much of a bother." Dr. Sheri agrees. "What's one more shot when you've had thousands in your lifetime? They usually don't hurt much anyway."

What makes insulin delivery even easier today is that there is a variety of ways to deliver it as well, including using "pens," insulin pumps, and inhaled insulins. The pens hold prefilled insulin cartridges, and the desired insulin dose is "dialed in" prior to being injected. As Blondie Fram says, "Insulin pens are wonderful. I don't use syringes anymore." For Peter Gariti, insulin pens have also made his life easier. "They're so easy to carry around in my shirt pocket," he says, "and I think they're more accurate." He uses separate pens for both his Lantus and his NovoLog doses. As for insulin pumps, they require one needle stick (when the infusion set is inserted) once every three to five days for most people, and then all of the insulin during that time is directly infused into the skin through that catheter. Many people enjoy having to worry less about injections while still getting their insulin over those few days. Likewise, inhaled insulins are simply breathed in using measured doses (which works well unless you have some pulmonary issues like asthma or frequent colds), but their absorption is not yet as precise as injected varieties.

Using insulin pens can also reduce the likelihood of giving yourself a dose of the wrong insulin when you use more than one (and many of the vials look similar) because each insulin has its own unique injection pen. By way of example, all it took was Dr. Sheri mistakenly giving her evening dose of Lantus (six units) as an equivalent amount of Humalog one time before she switched to using a Lantus pen to avoid making that type of error again. (Just for your information, to cover an extra six-unit dose of rapid-acting insulin when she normally only takes two for dinner, Dr. Sheri had to eat about twenty-five marshmallows, four graham crackers, six glucose tablets, and a few more items just to keep from bottoming out, and then she ended up nearly 400 mg/dl in the middle of the night when all of the food was finally digested.)

Oftentimes when older individuals develop a form of type 1 called latent autoimmune diabetes of the adult, or LADA, their insulin needs are low for several years, and they may be misdiagnosed as having type 2. Most individuals with type 1, however, will require insulin from the start, and oral medications will not effectively treat their condition. The worst thing to do with a child with rapid-onset type 1 is to put him or her on oral medications instead, since going on insulin immediately will help preserve the remaining insulin-making beta cells and keep the "honeymoon" going longer. On occasion, though, type 1 children have also been misdiagnosed and mistreated. For instance, when Anna Maria Gould was diagnosed with diabetes back in the mid-1960s at the age of 9, her doctor at the time put her on oral medications for the first two years. She remained "skinny and scrawny" on that regimen even though her mother was trying hard to keep her controlled, until she finally went into a diabetic coma caused by hyperglycemia, at which point the doctor in the emergency room (a different one) asked, "Why isn't this child on insulin?" Once she was treated properly with insulin injections, she finally got her blood sugars under better control and gained some weight back.

For people with type 2 diabetes, taking oral medications is equally as important (see table). Several older classes of oral medications are also still used. Metformin (sold as Glucophage and generic products) mainly targets the liver to reduce its blood glucose production overnight and after meals. If your fasting glucose levels are typically high, this drug is usually prescribed. Sulfonylureas like Amaryl and Glyburide help stimulate your pancreas to make more insulin (as long as it's able to). Both Actos and Avandia, drugs in the thiazolidinedione (TZD) class, work by sensitizing fat and muscle cells to insulin. Although the safety of Avandia, in particular with regard to heart health, has recently been questioned, this drug remains on the market. Combination drugs that combine two of these classes of drugs together, such as Avandia and Amaryl to form Avandaryl, are catching on, since it makes taking multiple drugs (often necessary for effective control of type 2 diabetes) easier.

ORAL AND OTHER DIABETIC MEDICATIONS

Class of Drug	Examples (Brand Name)	Mechanism of Action(s)
Sulfonylureas	Amaryl, DiaBeta, Diabinese, Glynase, Micronase	Promote insulin secretion from the beta cells of the pancreas; some may increase insulin sensitivity.
Thiazolidenediones "Glitazones"	Avandia, Actos	Increase insulin sensitivity of peripheral tissues, such as muscle.
Biguanides	Glucophage, Glucophage XR, Riomet, Glumetza, metformin (generic)	Decrease liver glucose muscle insulin sensitivity; output; increase liver and no direct effect on beta cells.
Meglitinides/ phenylalanine derivatives	Prandin, Starlix	Stimulate beta cells to increase insulin secretion, but only for a very short duration (unlike sulfonylureas).
Alpha-glucosidase inhibitors	Precose, Glyset	Work in intestines to slow digestion of some carbohydrates to control post-meal blood glucose peaks.
Amylin	Symlin (injected)	Works in combination with insulin to control glycemic spikes for three hours after meals.
Incretins	Byetta (injected)	Stimulate insulin release; inhibit the liver's release of glucose via glucagon; delay the emptying of food from the stomach.
DDP-4 inhibitors	Januvia, Galvus (seeking FDA approval)	Work by inhibiting DPP-4, an enzyme that breaks down glucagon-like peptide-1 (GLP-1); delayed GLP-1 degradation extends the action of insulin while suppressing glucagon release.

Type 2 diabetes tends to be a progressive disease, and the medications that used to control the condition may stop working after a while. In Robert Mandell's experience, "Anyone on pills for diabetes, if he or she lives long enough, will end up on insulin." In his case, he didn't even need pills for his first 15 years with diabetes because he was so diligent with his dietary changes and exercise routine. When he finally started taking oral medications, his doctor kept changing his pills because they stopped working effectively over time (a very common occurrence in anyone with type 2). Finally, he started requiring twice-daily doses of NPH insulin in the past six to seven years. Having to supplement with insulin doesn't mean that you're a failure, though. Type 2 diabetes can cause a progressive loss of pancreatic beta cells, and if you live long enough with this disease, these insulin-producing cells may simply give out after a while, particularly if your blood glucose control is not equivalent to that of anyone without diabetes.

32

Love (or Hate) Your Pump

Whether you have type 1 or type 2 diabetes, if you use insulin, you may choose to give it to yourself using a specialized insulin pump, which nowadays is about the size of a pager or cell phone. Pumps utilize a subcutaneous catheter through which small, basal doses of short-acting insulin are continually delivered to mimic normal insulin release by the pancreas. You also

THE LATEST AND GREATEST INSULIN PUMPS

Made By	Latest Models
Medtronic MiniMed, Inc.	Paradigm 522 and 722
Animas Corporation	IR 1250 and newer 2020
Smiths Medical MD, Inc.	CozMore Insulin Technology System
Insulet Corporation	OmniPod
Roche (formerly Disetronic Medical Systems Inc.)	Accu-Chek Spirit
Sooil USA	Dana Diabecare II, S, and SG
Nipro Diabetes Systems	Amigo

Noteworthy Features	More Information
Pumps and real-time continuous glucose monitor can be used together (one screen for both).	www.minimed.com, (800) 933-3322
Smallest basal increments of 0.025 units; automatic bolus calculator; EzCarb 500-item carb content list, and high-contrast color screen (2020 only).	www.animascorp.com, (877) 937-7867
All-in-one pump (Deltec Cozmo) and glucose monitor (FreeStyle); free CoZManager software; AAA batteries.	www.cozmore.com, (800) 826-9703
Disposable (3 days); no tubing; wireless Personal Diabetes Manager; integrated Freestyle meter; easy cannula insertion.	www.myomnipod.com, (800) 591-3455
Comes with free glucose meter and Palm PDA for bolus calculations and easy carb counting.	www.disetronic-usa.com, (800) 280-7801
Extremely small and lightweight; 20% lower retail price; preset meal boluses; built-in glucose meter (SG model).	www.danapumps.com, (858) 404-0659
Built-in bolus estimator (no manual calculations).	www.niprodiabetes.com, (888) 651-7867

must program the pump to give yourself bolus doses to cover your food (mainly carbohydrate) intake at meals and snacks. The idea behind insulin pump therapy is to provide insulin just like your body would—in small doses all day long, with bigger doses following food ingestion. While this same physiological pattern can be closely mimicked using any of the newer basal/bolus regimens (e.g., Lantus insulin for basal, Humalog or NovoLog for boluses), insulin pumps make the delivery of that insulin easier, and they offer more flexibility by allowing the user to change basal rates of insulin delivery at any time during the day.

Many different insulin pumps are now available, and the features vary by manufacturer and model. Most of the manufacturers' respective pumps nowadays have features such as small basal increments (0.05 units per hour or less), temporary basal rates, menu-driven programming, and various bolus patterns (e.g., normal, extended, and combination). At least two even have self-contained food databases or blood glucose meters, and most are now waterproof at shallow depths. With all these options, it can be hard to decide which pump to get, so you may want to talk to your health-care provider after going to each manufacturer's Web site or calling for more information. Some special features of each are listed in the table that follows. You can also research and compare various models on your own either online at the Diabetes Mall (www.diabetesnet.com/diabetes_technology/insulin_pump_models.php) or Children with Diabetes (www.childrenwithdiabetes.com/pumps/links.htm), or by getting a copy of the annual spring issue of *Diabetes Health* magazine (www.DiabetesHealth.com), which provides an extremely comprehensive pump feature comparison guide.

A new self-contained, disposable insulin pump called the OmniPod was one of the latest (and most revolutionary) ones to hit the market. Its primary selling point is that the pumps are disposable after every three days of wear; they also require no exogenous tubing, given that all of the insulin is self-contained in the pump itself, which you program to deliver the insulin using a separate, handheld control unit. Don Gifford uses one, but he states, "I am not as big a fan of it than of the DexCom [a continuous glucose-monitoring device discussed in Secret 35]. Pods are nice as long as you don't lose the control unit. Also, sometimes they fall off; they tend to take up more space than normal infusion sets; and there are fewer sites possible to put them." Dr. Steve also uses an OmniPod pump, which he likes primarily because of its tubing-free design.

Insulin pumps can be both a blessing and a curse, however, and the choice of whether to use one or not should be an individual one. Of the more than fifty interviewees for this book, slightly more than half of them are "pumpers." After living with type 2 diabetes for over 18 years, Zach Barneis went on an insulin pump about five years ago, and he says, "It changed my life completely." Carol Sessions, Chuck Eichten, and Barbara Baxter all report no longer having bad bouts of hypoglycemia since they started using pumps. As Barbara comments, "It really has been a blessing, and I wish I had gone on it sooner." Bernadette McIntyre echoes her sentiments: "I only went on a pump five or six years ago, but I wish now that I had gone on it sooner. I was getting more brittle, but was stubborn and vain. Luckily, my cousin talked me into it." For Anna Maria Gould, insulin pumps have worked well for her for the past eight or more years. She finds them easier to use because she doesn't have to continually balance her long- and short-acting insulins.

Freddi Fredrickson obviously likes pumping as well, given that she has been using an insulin pump for the past 27 years, since they first came on the market in 1980. John Rodosevich is another one of those people who loves his pump. "I've been on a pump since 1982," he says. "It has definitely improved my quality of life, and I'm very happy with it." He also thinks that people on pumps are generally self-motivated, gregarious, and outgoing. Jane Dohrmann is another "pumper" who has been using one for over a decade. She says, "Switching from multiple injections to an insulin pump in 1996 was the best move I have ever made. I am able to fine-tune my control so much easier now."

For Marialice Kern, going on a pump is one of her top secrets for longevity with diabetes. "I haven't had any bad lows since going on a pump, and my sensitivity to lows has come back." She also credits her pump with helping to preserve her kidney function. She decided to start using one after having a car accident resulting from undetected hypoglycemia, as did Bill King. At that point, Bill's wife said to him, "You need to get your act together." He researched the two main pump manufacturers at the time (Disetronic and MiniMed), finally deciding to go on the former pump. For him, its impact was most remarkable when it came to exercising: He found that by manipulating the basal rates, he could actually go running and not develop hypoglycemia like he used to when using insulin injections that included intermediate-acting insulins like NPH.

Chuck Eichten is equally excited about his pump. "When I first went on a pump over five years ago," he says, "I was astounded at how effective it was and wondered why no one had told me before how viable a treatment it is." He also wondered if he was the last person to go on one (we can assure him that he's not). For him, being on a pump has also stopped him from having additional hypoglycemia-induced seizures, which he had started to have on a regular basis when he was on his NPH and Regular insulin regimen. "Everyone gets so excited about the technology, but for me it's really all just about having a better lifestyle."

It's true that a pump is only as good as the person in charge of it, though. Insulin pumps are usually filled with a rapid-acting insulin (or Regular, although using this insulin in a pump is less favored due to its later peak and longer duration), so if the pump stops delivering basal insulin for any reason, you can soon find yourself in DKA, even within just a few hours. Anna Maria Gould reminds us, "You have to always be aware of what's going on with your pump. It's a machine, and it's up to you to control it."

Although many old-timers swear by insulin pumps, others have experienced more limitations with them, refused to use them, or tried and given up on them. Mary Sue Rubin states that although her pump has been good for her (she has been using one since 1983), it also has caused some problems. She was one of the first three people in Baltimore to go on a pump all those years ago, but her first pump leaked at the luer-lock connection (where the tubing connects to the syringe containing the reservoir of insulin), and she has additionally experienced getting bubbles in the infusion line when using some of the older infusion sets. As she notes, a pump at this point in time is only as good as the person wearing it, although she admits, "At times, I get a little sloppy; I get distracted and forget to bolus."

Dick Bernstein, who manages the care of many people with all types of diabetes, believes that most people do better off of insulin pumps because of the potentially negative impact of having an indwelling foreign body (the infusion set catheter) continually under the skin. "Being on a pump doesn't necessarily help your blood sugar control, except in comparison to only taking one to two shots a day," he says. In his opinion, using a pump is no better than doing multiple daily injections. For example, Paul McGuigan used an insulin pump for ten years while he was involved as a subject in the "intensive treatment" group for the Diabetes Control and Complications Trial (DCCT), but a decade ago when he was at the summer camp for diabetic kids that he's involved with, he took it off because a lot of the kids back then didn't have one. So far, he has never gone back to using one, but he feels that his control is the same.

It's actually quite common to develop significant scar tissue at the infusion sites, which can make it harder for your insulin to be effectively delivered. "After five years on a pump, I had a lot of scar tissue on my abdomen where I put all of my infusion sets," says Dr. Sheri. "For that reason, I decided to go on a 'pump vacation' six years ago that I'm still enjoying." After more than 25 years on an insulin pump, Karen Poenisch has just found alternate scar-tissue-free spots to use instead, such as under her arms and on the sides of her breasts. "If you have enough extra padding, you can find lots of spots to use," she admits.

❦ 33 ❧

Find Out the Benefits of Newer Medications

The new millennium has brought the first approval of a newer drug to treat type 1 diabetes in over 80 years (since the discovery of insulin in 1921). This new medication is called Symlin, and it is a synthetic form of the body's natural hormone, amylin, which is normally released from the beta cells of the pancreas simultaneously with insulin. Matt Besley, who works for Amylin Pharmaceuticals, contends that "the biggest barrier to good diabetes control is that the disease requires more than one hormone, and we've only been treating it with one hormone all these years." Rabbi Meisels adds, "The problem that Symlin addresses is important, and we can't ignore it anymore." Karen Poenisch, Dr. Steve, Larry Verity, and others find that it blunts their after-meal highs, which has shown to be important for preventing complications in both type 1 and type 2 diabetes. Dick Bernstein contends that this hormone can help people control their snacking, if nothing else.

One drawback of Symlin use is that this synthetic form of amylin must be injected like insulin. Its main action is to work with insulin following meals to control the flow of glucose coming from the food that you ate into your circulation. If you have to inject insulin to control your post-meal highs, then your body likely is not releasing enough of this hormone naturally. The main side effects of the synthetic, supplemental form are the potential for severe hypoglycemia (the risk is greater in all insulin users), nausea, vomiting, abdominal pain, headache, fatigue, and dizziness. Both of us know individuals who have tried Symlin but stopped because they couldn't handle the nausea it caused. For instance, Rabbi Meisels found that he could only tolerate much less than the recommended doses (about one unit instead of the recommended 2.5). He alternately tried infusing it at a rate of 0.5 units per hour using a second (insulin) pump, and although his glucose excursions were more controlled, he ultimately stopped because the hassle of wearing two pumps was, in his words, "a little too much."

A potential additional benefit is that Symlin can help you lose some weight, possibly due to tighter blood sugar control and feelings of fullness sooner during a meal. For example, Bill King has found that using Symlin together with insulin boluses helps him correct his blood sugars more rapidly when he becomes hyperglycemic following a big meal. As an added benefit, it may also reduce oxidative stress and prevent you from developing diabetic complications, although this potential effect needs to be further studied. However, if you have gastroparesis, you may not want to use this medication routinely because it can cause more frequent, severe hypoglycemia by further slowing your already less rapid absorption of food. You may also want to be careful about taking it before exercise sessions, as it can make exercise-induced hypo-glycemia harder to treat by slowing the absorption of any glucose or food you take to raise your low sugars. Several athletes that Dr. Sheri knows have complained about getting "Symlin lows" that they couldn't get out of easily following exercise.

Another new medication made by the manufacturers of Symlin is Byetta, a new injectable medication that is mainly intended for the treatment of type 2 diabetes, although some people with slow-onset type 1 in adulthood have used it to try to regenerate some of their insulin-producing beta cells. It may also have some benefits for type 1s who are more insulin resistant. In some ways, Byetta acts like Symlin, causing food to empty from the stomach more slowly and glucose levels to stay lower after meals. It also stimu-lates the pancreas to make more insulin, which is an effect that would not benefit most type 1s. It also keeps the liver from over-producing glucose, and in most users, it results in weight loss. This new class of medications effectively replaces natural hormones normally released by the digestive tract ("gut hormones") after meals to spur insulin release and provides another choice for dia-betes treatment, particularly if your treatment with oral diabetic medications is no longer working effectively. A drawback, though, is that it has to be injected (rather than ingested) twice a day, which may not be that desirable to anyone who hasn't gone on insulin to avoid taking shots. Some additional classes of new med-ications for people with type 2 diabetes are also in the pipeline for future release that also target insulin release and insulin action, including Januvia (already available) and Galvus, both of which work with gut hormones, natural enzymes, and the body's own insulin to control blood glucose levels.

In one case, an old medication may have found a new use. A recent study investigated the use of Glucophage in overweight adults with type 1 diabetes, even though this drug is normally only prescribed to treat type 2. This oral antidiabetic medication approved for use by the FDA in 1994 actually has multiple actions, working to decrease the liver's production of new glucose (gluconeogenesis), lower glucose absorption from the gut, and increase insulin sensitivity around the body. To our knowledge, it has not been prescribed in normal weight type 1s, but it may prove to be a useful therapy in overweight individuals with type 1 diabetes who have started to exhibit a reduced insulin action more common to type 2 diabetes.

❧ 34 ❧

Explore the Latest Technology

Blood glucose meters have come a long way in the past two-plus decades, but then again, most people who have lived a long time with diabetes remember back to when testing for sugar in your urine was the only method for trying to estimate your blood sugars at home (although you still never knew what they really were). "It was a totally different world then," says Jim Arthur. He remembers having to get his blood taken at the doctor's office at each visit, but then having to wait two or more weeks to get the test results.

All of the people with diabetes for longer than 20 years remember these bad ol' days of urine testing. Originally, the testing involved boiling Benedict's solution in a test tube over a Bunsen burner or stove, but later progressed to the urine testing that Dr. Sheri started out with: putting five drops of urine plus ten drops of water in a test tube, adding a Clinitest tablet, and watching it react and boil up in the test tube. All the while, you'd be praying, "Come on, blue . . . come on, blue," because a blue color indicated a lack of sugar in the urine. If any was present though (and it usually starts spilling over into the urine when you exceed your renal threshold, which is around 200 mg/dl for most people), the boiling and bubbling concoction would turn different shades ranging from green (trace) to bright orange (4+, meaning a whole lot of sugar was in it).

As a kid, Dr. Sheri remembers what negative feedback it was for the solution to bubble up bright orange so often. "I felt like I was doing something wrong all the time," she says. "I could be in the middle of a hypoglycemic reaction, and it would still indicate a '4+' level of sugar." Urine testing was time-delayed, since the urine had to be produced and excreted, which could be several hours after your body made it. In the mornings, you were supposed to do a double void (that is, urinating, waiting about fifteen minutes, and catching a sample to test the second), which was supposed to give you a sample of more recently made urine for better accuracy, if you could really call any urine testing "accurate." As Natalie Saunders shares, "With urine testing, I was almost always 4+ even though I was doing everything right. It was very discouraging."

Patty Schaeffer even remembers how urine testing was used to diagnose her diabetes back in 1937 when she was only three and a half years old. "I have a vivid memory of the urine test done in the doctor's office. As I recall it, the room where the testing was done was dark, except for bright lights that were in the lab area where the urine testing was done, and I saw it turn bright orange." When Julie Krupnick was diagnosed with diabetes at the age of 12 back in 1979, she remembers one particular urine testing incident. When her urine test remained blue one morning not long after her diagnosis, she thought she didn't have diabetes anymore and told her mother so. "Let me get you some break-fast," she recalls her mother replying. Jim Turner expressed his frustration with this form of testing thus: "After two years of urine testing, I decided it wasn't telling me anything. I just got my blood glucose tested once every three to four months."

"I'm sure my blood sugar control was not very good until I had a blood glucose meter," Bob Elder voices for himself and the rest of us old-timers, along with Karen Poenisch, who says, "Who knows what our blood sugar was back then?" A 41-year diabetes veteran, Jane Dohrmann was thrilled when she would be able to start testing her blood sugars at home with an actual monitor, once they were available. "I would no longer have to use those poisonous tablets, pee in a cup, and pretend to be a scientist, adding so many drops of pee and so many drops of water, knowing that the value I was going to get still wasn't going to be accurate."

Early prototypes of home glucose monitors were bulky and expensive. The first one that Dick Bernstein had back in the 1970s was as big as a textbook, and Marc Blatstein remembers having one that large as well. Grant McArthur recalls that his first meter was the size of a small book and took a long time to use. "You had to program it for every strip," he remembers. "It was hard to use." They were also quite pricey, making them a luxury that most people at that time just couldn't afford.

Today's meters, though, are inexpensive and a joy to use, and you can choose the one with the features you like. Most of us old-timers, who went through a number of years without knowing what our blood sugars were, are just happy having the opportunity to check our blood sugars, since knowing what they actually are has made all the difference in the world. (It's just an added bonus that it only takes about five seconds to find out what your blood sugar is nowadays.) Most insulin users test anywhere from four to fifteen or more times a day. "Now, they're small and easy to use," comments Grant McArthur about meters, "although they would be expensive to use without insurance coverage to cover the strips." He's right on that count. The initial investment in the meters is relatively minimal, but even with insurance reimbursement, most of us end up paying at least twenty cents a strip. You can't put a price tag on the value of knowing what your blood sugars are, though. For most of us, paying any amount is more than worth it to preserve our good health.

Matt Besley says one of his main secrets is to always explore new technology to try to improve glucose control, including newer blood glucose monitor and other tools. "You may not always like what you try," he says, "but at least try new things." He also advises people to find a doctor who is interested in trying them out, too. As for Peter Gariti, he thinks that living with diabetes is a lot more trouble-free now than it used to be when he was diagnosed 60 years ago. "People may think it's difficult to have diabetes now," he remarks, "but it's so much easier to control your blood sugars now. If the advances keep coming like they have been, it'll just get easier and easier to have a good quality of life with diabetes and to stay alive." Jane Dohrmann comments, "My mom used to call it being 'nosey,' but my inquisitiveness is how I have learned new things about the changes that have taken place with diabetes technology and care." Regardless of what you call it, we feel that it's a trait that serves people with diabetes well. "Now all we need is a noninvasive blood glucose-monitoring system," says Jim Arthur. "Then everyone would be happy and everything would be right with the world." Just wait a little longer, Jim; they're working on it as you read.

✤ 35 ✤

Monitor Continuously

The first continuous glucose monitors to be approved by the FDA finally hit the market in 2006 and took off running even though they're still invasive, requiring a probe placed under your skin. These monitors are not a "closed-loop" system either, meaning that you still have to see the blood glucose readings and make regimen adjustments yourself, but getting readings every five minutes or more twenty-four hours a day can be extremely useful to people trying to keep their blood glucose in good control (like all of the long-time diabetes survivors and hopefully you).

The four continuous glucose-monitoring (CGM) models currently available include the DexCom STS, the Medtronic MiniMed Guardian RT and Paradigm Real-Time System, and the Abbott FreeStyle Navigator. Insurance reimbursement is hit-or-miss, depending on the insurance provider and the individual's overall diabetes care needs. All of these models vary in price, with start-up costs ranging from $800 for DexCom (although they often run new-user specials) to more than $2,000 (for the Medtronic MiniMed Guardian) for the transmitters, receivers, a set of sensors, and other necessary supplies. The individual sensors are similar in price among the four, about $35 each, undoubtedly with better insurance coverage to come in the near future. They all have user-set high and low alarms, insertion devices, associated computer software to manage data, and similar accuracy, but only the Abbott monitor has a built-in Freestyle glucose meter. (Check out more of their features in the following table.) All are considered "durable medical equipment," which is

SPECIFIC FEATURES OF THE FOUR CURRENTLY AVAILABLE CONTINUOUS MONITORING SYSTEMS

	Abbott Freestyle Navigator
FDA-approved sensor life	5 days
Glucose results displayed on insulin pump?	No
Length of sensor probe and insertion angle	6 mm, 90 degrees
Start-up initialization	10 hours
Calibration	Calibrate at 10, 12, 24, and 72 hours, with no more calibrations for the final 2 days of the 5-day wear
Frequency of readings	Every minute
Display of directional trends?	Yes, directional and rate of change arrows; 2, 4 ,6, 12, or 24 hour glucose graph; can go back 28 days
Transmitter waterproof?	Yes
Monitor-to-transmitter range	10 feet (but possibly more)
Sensor storage	4 months at room temperature
Transmitter batteries	Watch battery; replace monthly
Monitor batteries	2 AAA batteries; replace every 3 months

Medtronic MiniMed Paradigm Real-Time System	Medtronic MiniMed Guardian RT	DexCom STS
3 days	3 days	3 (original) and 7 (newer ones) days
Yes, using Paradigm 522 and 722 pumps, CGM on pump screen	No	No
13 mm, 45 degrees	13 mm, 45 degrees	13 mm, 45 degrees
2 hours	2 hours	2 hours
At 2 hours, again within 6 hours, and then every 12 hours	At 2 hours, again within 6 hours, and then every 12 hours	Must calibrate with LifeScan One Touch Ultra, two times to start, then at least once every 12 hours
Every 5 minutes	Every 5 minutes	Every 5 minutes
Yes, arrows display how fast and in what direction, plus 3- and 24-hour graphs	No, must manually scroll; can upload data to software for analysis	Yes, displays 1-, 3-, or 9-hour glucose graphs
Yes, up to 8 feet deep for 30 minutes	Yes, up to 8 feet deep for 30 minutes	No, but shower patch makes watertight
6 feet	6 feet	5 feet
6 months refrigerated, 1 week at room temperature	6 months refrigerated, 1 week at room temperature	4 months at room temperature
Nonreplaceable; 9-month life	Nonreplaceable; 12-month life	Nonreplaceable; 6-month warranty
No separate monitor; results displayed on pump	2 AAA batteries; alerts when replacement needed	Must recharge the battery every 5 days, charge time 3 hours

not returnable after you open the box they come in (although the transmitters can be returned for a limited amount of time).

The CGM systems recently approved for use in the United States are admittedly "first-generation" products, meaning that they're likely to improve when newer versions come out, just like blood glucose meters and insulin pumps have enhanced their technology with each new model (see table). "Continuous glucose monitoring is like testing with a meter was in the 1980s when you first got one," comments Karen Poenisch. "You can use them to see if you're matching your food and your insulin right, and you can see what happens when you eat fat. They have the potential to have an extremely positive effect on a person's control."

So far, people either love or hate these monitors. Dr. Steve has been wearing a DexCom sensor almost since the unit came on the market in April 2006, and he wouldn't want to be without it. However, Dr. Sheri tried one for about three weeks and then gave up using it. "Its trends weren't even right," she complains. "I was ending up checking my blood sugars all of the time—at least twice as many times as I normally do—because I never knew whether to believe the numbers or not." Although Dr. Steve and others have found their sensors to track correctly for them about 80 percent of the time, Dr. Sheri was lucky if her numbers were close about half of the time. "I woke up low one night, really low and shaking like a leaf. I usually just treat it, since I know I'm low, but because the DexCom said I was 130, I tested to see how far it was off. I was down to 42 mg/dl." Dr. Steve still sees these devices becoming a standard of diabetes care, though. He says, "Be patient and have realistic expectations. The current continuous monitors are first-generation devices, and you may have technical problems, but the technical support people are friendly and ready to help. We have been waiting for continuous glucose monitoring for a long time, and these devices will only get better with time." Dr. Sheri agrees with his statement about the ease and availability of technical support, at least as far as her DexCom experiences are concerned.

For Don Gifford, a professor of law at the University of Maryland, wearing the DexCom CGMS has allowed him to be better controlled now than ever. "I usually bounced between 60 and 220, but I rarely hit that high now. I'm usually between 70 and 200 using the DexCom." Matt Besley agrees that the DexCom helps him to figure out the best timing of his insulin and Symlin injections. "It's better as a trending tool, though," he admits.

Carol Sessions says hypoglycemia is her biggest barrier to good diabetes control, but getting the DexCom system has helped a lot. She has been using an insulin pump for a quarter of a century already (since 1982) and counts her carbs, but she is able to adjust her insulin more effectively with the DexCom, and it also allows her to see her glycemic trends at night. In fact, she's learning even more about the effects of the foods she eats by being able to see her body's immediate reaction to them. "It may take a year for me to hit all the major holidays with the DexCom," she says.

Bernadette McIntyre is also very excited about having a Medtronic continuous glucose-monitoring device that can display her CGM results on her Medtronic insulin pump. "I still check my blood sugar a lot of times during the day, but at a quick glance, it gives me a good idea how my blood sugar are responding. I'm using it to figure out if my pump's basal rates are correct, since I don't like skipping meals." Although Marialice Kern enjoyed using the DexCom during a clinical trial she participated in, she is also going to get the Medtronic MiniMed Paradigm Real-Time System (that will display both pump and CGM information on her pump's screen) once her insurance covers it.

You may even be able to use continuous-monitoring results to better motivate you and help you make better decisions about your care. Take Freddi Fredrickson, for example, who says, "What

I really love about having a continuous monitor is that when I look and see that my blood sugar is a little high, I can say 'no, thanks' to dessert." She also admits that she feels a sense of security when she is in a normal range, particularly since she worries about getting low more than high. Bill King also says, "Using a continuous glucose monitor like the DexCom encourages you to check your blood sugar more often." He agrees that it's frustrating to have a sensor that gives less accurate results than is desirable, but he loves having the ones that track his sugars well. In the immediate future, continuous glucose monitoring will likely be an invaluable aid to help people get better control over their diabetes by learning their glycemic trends. "Thanks to all the advances in diabetes care," says Bernadette McIntyre, "I look forward to living fully and well in the future."

Some people have gotten their sensors to give readings for up to twenty-six days straight, but more often than not, they're only good for three to seven days. "Some of mine didn't even last that long," says Dr. Sheri. "I'm going to wait for the next-generation product and until my health insurance company decides to start covering at least a portion of its costs." Eventually, devices like the continuous glucose-monitoring ones are bound to get more and more accurate and be able to mesh with an insulin pump to create an artificial pancreas of sorts. In all likelihood, we're at least 10 to 15 years away from that possibility, though. In the meantime, try one out if you want to, and see what you can learn from knowing what your blood sugars are doing all of the time. Many old-timers have still learned new things about how to better control their diabetes using the latest technology, and if you think you will be able to learn anything from using one, then it's probably still worth a try, even given its current limitations of having less-than-optimal accuracy all of the time and being expensive to use. If your control is already excellent, though, you may not see many improvements coming from wearing a continuous monitor.

❧ 36 ❧

Check Out Clinical Trials

Many long-living people with diabetes have kept on the cutting edge of diabetes treatments and technologies by getting involved in clinical trials of new medical devices and medications. For instance, Paul McGuigan got involved in the clinical trials called the Diabetes Control and Complications Trial (DCCT) from nearly the beginning of his time with diabetes. He's also been in the long-term follow-up trials. As a consequence, he has been receiving excellent treatment for his diabetes almost the entire time he has had the disease. "I have always had pretty good control because I was in the DCCT from the start," he says. "For the first ten years, my A1c was never above 7.8 percent, and I've maintained the same or better since the trial ended. What with the study's follow-up, I've been involved with it for 22 years now. Luckily, I was randomized into the intensive treatment arm and put on a pump during the study."

Bill King benefited similarly from being in the same intensive treatment arm of the DCCT at another study site in Pennsylvania. "I got into the DCCT three and a half years after my diagnosis," he says. "They did all sorts of testing on me, so I knew they were looking at the benefits of good control. Being in the DCCT had a significant impact on me because it taught me how to achieve good control and the importance of intensive diabetes management." He said the bigger problem was continuing to achieve that level of control after the study ended, this time on his own. "They sent us on our way when the study ended with the thought that we were going to be able to stay intensively managed." It wasn't as easy, but at least when he would have a run of bad control afterward, he could use what he had learned as motivation to get back on track.

Typically, clinical trials are divided into phases, depending on what stage the medication or therapy has reached. For example, phase I trials are all about whether the treatment is safe. Usually, only a small number of volunteers are involved, and different doses of a medication may be tried out while monitoring for side effects occurs. Phase II are more about efficacy, or how well the treatment works; this phase involves testing a larger number of people. The next phase (III) takes place as long as the second phase showed the treatment to be effective and without excessive side effects. This phase involves hundreds to many thousands of people and further tests the treatment's effectiveness. Oftentimes, the new treatment will be tested against any existing ones. Finally, phase IV trials are conducted after the new product has received approval from the FDA and made it onto the market. Thus, its main purpose is to look for any new side effects in a larger group of people that might not have been detected in the third phase, along with testing alternate uses of the medication or therapy.

HOW TO GET INVOLVED IN DIABETES-RELATED RESEARCH TRIALS

You can find out more information about diabetes-related research trials on the American Diabetes Association's Web site: www.diabetes.org/diabetes-research/clinical-trials/trials-home.jsp. To find ongoing trials that you can join, try searching online for ones in your area at Veritas Medicine for Patients, found at www.veritasmedicine.com. In addition, the National Institutes of Health (NIH) provides general information about clinical trials and a search service accessible at www.clinicaltrials.gov, which allows you to type in the medical condition (such as "diabetes" or "neuropathy") or treatment (e.g., "inhaled insulin" or "continuous glucose monitors") along with your location to find nearby trials for which you might qualify. Finally, many related to type 1 diabetes only are listed on the Juvenile Diabetes Research Foundation's Web site, which you can find at www.jdrf.org/index.cfm?page_id=101984.

There are many potential benefits associated with getting involved in clinical trials. Doing so may be the best way to get exposed to the latest and greatest in diabetes care before it's available to the public at large. Many individuals have tried out continuous blood glucose monitors, Symlin, and other treatments through their involvement. By way of example, Marialice Kern was in a clinical trial of the DexCom continuous glucose monitor before it received FDA approval, and she has more recently been in a trial of their second-generation, seven-day sensors. Besides exposing you to cutting-edge technologies and treatment options, being in a clinical trial means that you get to participate at no cost. Given how much the continuous glucose-monitoring sensors are going for on the market (and with only a select group of people currently with insurance to cover them), we would all be smart to volunteer for as many clinical trials in our area as we can. Also, invariably you will have greater access to health-care professionals and cost-free medical advice while you're involved in a clinical trial—primarily because such trials can have untoward side effects, which is the main downside of participating. Some people participate in clinical trials to contribute to medical science and to help doctors and researchers find better ways to help others, if not themselves. In any case, participation in trials is completely voluntary, and you will be apprised of the possible risks and benefits before you ever agree to participate.

DOLORES "DEE" BREHM, AGE 77, LIVING WITH TYPE 1 DIABETES FOR 58 YEARS

When Dee Brehm was diagnosed in 1949 with type 1 diabetes, her prospects were not bright: a permanent chronic condition, a reduced life span, potentially devastating complications, and perhaps no children. She married Bill Brehm in 1952, and they began a partnership knowing that together they would have to manage her disease. Now, Dee is defying that dim outlook for her life: She has two children and six grandchildren, she has surpassed the half-century mark with this disease, and she has been spared the ordeal of complications.

Diagnosed at 19, Dee was then attending college in Michigan and had to assume full responsibility for her day-to-day care at a time when care was a challenge, as the tools were primitive: Her glass syringes had to be boiled and their needles sharpened on emery cloth, and the only means of measuring her blood sugar was a urine test that required a near chemistry lab process.

Dee, now a resident of McLean, Virginia, says, "I was blessed with having a committed husband and partner in my diabetes care all these years; I probably wouldn't be alive were it not for him. However, he is very careful not to take away my independence, although we stay in close communication, and I report my tests to him wherever he is. Together, we decide on the adjustments needed to respond to the inevitable lows and highs, as two heads are better than one in this business. His vigilance is vital in helping me control my disease."

The couple appears to be an unbeatable team. Some time after she passed the 50-year "gold-medal" milestone with diabetes, he asked her one evening when she was preparing dinner what he could do to help her. In response, she said, "You can find a cure." Bill was silent for a moment, and then simply said, "Okay."

With that goal in mind, the Brehms began an odyssey in 1999 to learn about the work being done to cure diabetes, which ultimately led to their making a proposal to the University of Michigan to create a center devoted to finding a cure for type 1. They donated $44 million of their own funds to make the center a reality and to apply new tools to facilitate the search process—most notably robust information science and systems analysis. Their goal is a cure in Dee's lifetime, which is to be accomplished through "a multifaceted, frontal assault" to determine the detailed causes of type 1 diabetes and how to cure it. Their approach depends heavily on collaboration and breaking down the administrative barriers that today inhibit rapid progress.

Despite being complication-free, Dee does not have an easy time with her diabetes. She tends to be brittle, causing her to constantly fear the onset of severe hypoglycemic episodes. To help her understand her trends and to determine adjustments in her program, she has kept meticulous records of her insulin doses and vital signs, including her weight and blood pressure. She is proud of her detailed records and notes that she has missed writing down a test result only once in 58 years. For her, discipline is key. Dee has taken well over 100,000 insulin injections and has tested her blood glucose over 65,000 times since first getting a glucose meter to use at home.

The Joslin Diabetes Center has undertaken a study of patients who have survived with type 1 for more than 50 years, of which there are likely only about 500 to 600 individuals in the United States who have been so fortunate. Some of those, like Dee, have not developed complications. Dee's records are an important part of the study, so all her attention to detail is paying off in ways that might help others. It is important to learn what has protected these people as that knowledge could contribute to the search for a cure. All in all, there is no question that all of us appreciate the efforts and devotion of this couple on behalf of all of those afflicted with type 1 diabetes.

PART SEVEN

Support Secrets

Always Ask for Help

Diabetes really is a team sport. You've heard the axiom, "It takes a village to raise a child," right? Along the same lines, "It takes a village to care for a diabetic," says Larry Verity. He says that you shouldn't be afraid to seek out help and support from others. In fact, it's useful to keep in mind that sometimes your diabetes can be harder on the people you live with than it is on you, and the more involved you allow them to be in your care, the more secure they may feel. Jim Arthur takes this principle to heart. "My wife gives me my morning injection in my butt where I can't reach, while I do the evening one in my stomach where I can." So does Gladys Dull, who let her husband give her shots when she ran out of places to give them to herself. "He gave them in my backside and other places I couldn't reach," she admits.

Marcy Shefsky of Newtown, Pennsylvania, insists that it's critical to let your coworkers and friends know that you have diabetes and how to help you if the need arises. "Let them know what to do or that they need to call someone for you if you're acting strange," she advises. Vena Petrotta agrees that it's important to get support from coworkers as well. Judy Tripathi also recommends, "Get guidance from others who really know how to steer you in the right direction." For Matt Besley, he thinks it's important to ask others to help you assess your progress. "Listen to the people around you. Ask them to give you feedback about what you're doing," he advises.

For Blondie Fram, assistance has been forthcoming from her family members for many years now. From the day she was widowed over 30 years ago (when she was in her late 50s), she has always lived with younger people, usually one of her daughters and occasionally her son and their respective families. For her, one of the most important aspects of doing well with type 2 diabetes for the past 40-plus years is having her children (and grandchildren) around to help her.

In the case of Jane Dohrmann, she admits to asking others for help on many occasions and feeling loyal to those who have helped her. "The people that have helped, guided, instructed, and cared for me all of these 40-plus years are important to me. Some are family members, some are friends, some are clinicians, and some have been strangers." She also says, "I would do anything for these people just to let them know how much I value them and appreciate them for everything they have done to help me to be so successful."

❦ 38 ❧

Seek Out Your Peers

Your diabetic peers are often the best source of information and support that there is. For instance, Freddi Fredrickson was in college when she was diagnosed. She didn't know anyone else with diabetes at all, so when she finally found out about another coed with it, she sought her out. "It felt so great to have a person similar to me to talk with—someone else with diabetes," she says. Likewise, one of Patty Schaeffer's secrets of diabetes longevity (70 years and counting) is to be involved with other people who know about or have diabetes. "Join groups," she advises. Patricia La France-Wolf agrees, and she tries to get the newly blind people in her classes to keep busy, stay socially connected, and go out with others, as well as to enroll in classes at the Braille Institute or senior centers near where they live outside of Pasadena, California. She belongs to a couple of blind diabetic groups herself and highly recommends them.

Many others have greatly benefited from the feedback of their diabetic peers as well. For instance, Barbara Baxter actually attended a pump support group for a year before deciding whether to go on a pump herself. She also strongly is in favor of going to support meetings of any kind. "They have been a big help," she states. "You can learn things from other people sharing their experiences." Rabbi Meisels says one of his secrets is to never assume that he knows it all. "You can always learn from others," he comments, "and even a small tip could make a big difference in your care." He also suggests joining a support group. In agreement with him, Jessica Ching says that finding your diabetic peers and talking to them, either in person or online, is key. In fact, for her it has been a lifesaver. Her internist had told her that she'd never be in good control, that there was no hope for her, and that she wasn't a good candidate for an insulin pump. Soon afterward, she volunteered for an ADA walk event and met someone there with an insulin pump, and her life changed forever on that day. She decided to switch doctors, went on an insulin pump (in 1991), and turned her life with diabetes around for the better.

John Rodosevich actually started an insulin pump support group himself back in 1982, and it still continues to meet to this day. He got the idea because there were five people he knew going to a weekly diabetes care management class at Kaiser Permanente back then, and they had lots of questions. When they talked with each other, they were amazed to find out what other people were doing that might benefit them. "I remember hanging my insulin pump on a coat hanger outside of the shower so it wouldn't get wet," John says. "I didn't realize until I talked to them that I could just disconnect it by removing the syringe." (Nowadays, all of the pumps disconnect from their infusion sets directly to allow you to take them off to shower, etc.) John also says that his pump support group has taken on a life of its own at this point. "We accept our role to help out new people coming for support, and a lot of meetings we devote to just helping one person by spending as much time as he or she needs. It's a very powerful experience when a group does that for you." The group consists of new- and old-timers, many of whom know so much and have so much to share with others. "There's a great satisfaction we all get from helping others," John admits. "It's good to be associated with people like that. They feel like family." To his credit, he also writes up a newsletter available to anyone who's interested.

Ron DeNunzio describes how important his diabetic peers have been to him. "I have two wonderful people who are type 1 diabetics, one that I have known for about ten years, the other for about three. They listen to me, and I listen to them," he says. "They have helped me in many ways. I got involved in 'My Diabetes' with their help and also the American Diabetes Association. I finally started doing things for diabetes and for myself. Through all this I have learned to take control of my diabetes."

Not all peer support has to occur in person, though. Nowadays, chat rooms and blogs on the Internet related to diabetes abound. One example is a diabetes chat room available through Children with Diabetes (www.childrenwithdiabetes.com/chat), which often allows young kids with diabetes themselves to "chat" with similar-aged peers (with adult supervision) at prescheduled times. There are even specific chat rooms for insulin pumpers (adults and children in various locations around the world), such as www.insulin-pumpers.org/chat.shtml and others. Take advantage of all of these resources to seek out help from other people in the know who might already know the answers to your burning questions about diabetes.

❧ 39 ❧

Involve Your Family and Friends

Most long-timers with diabetes agree that having a supportive husband, wife, significant other, family, and friends is a crucial secret to living well and long. In fact, studies have shown that connecting with others around you is one of the most important factors not only in avoiding depression, but also in reaching a higher level of happiness, which can keep you from stressing and overindulging in comfort foods that may raise your blood sugars (and make you feel guilty) or failing in your care in other ways.

Your family can be supportive in ways that are invaluable. For instance, Marcy Shefsky says that many times her kids will tell her that she's getting low blood sugar before she even realizes it, and she is not the only one who has this type of feedback and family support. During his 62 years of marriage to his wife Mildred, who passed away in 2002, Gerald Cleveland relied on her loving support. When she died, his daughter took over looking after him. She generally calls him in his retirement home at bedtime, 4:00 AM, and first thing in the morning to make sure that his blood sugars are not too low. "I really feel like I have had angels all around me," Gerald says. He has had his share of mishaps, though, many of them recent. He fell down when he was low fairly recently and split his forehead open, requiring eight stitches to fix. "Whenever I get into difficulty with my diabetes, someone or something is always there to help me." Even with this support, he feels a little down on occasion, sitting alone in his room. When he gets out with other people, he instantly feels supported, though.

"Marry a person who is willing and able to assist in your diabetes care," advises Patty Schaeffer. She credits her husband's assistance as being an integral part of her avoidance of bad low blood sugar reactions for the past eight years. Gladys Dull says, "I never thought I'd get married because of my diabetes. When we met, my husband said it didn't make a difference to him." He was continually supportive of his wife during their 59-year marriage that ended with his death in 2002. Vena Petrotta also acknowledges how critical the support of those closest to her has been over the years. "First it was my parents, now my daughters. I even had 38 years of support from my husband." Jim Arthur also raves about the help his wife has given him during 49 of his 64 years with diabetes. "She's my primary care provider," he says proudly. "She couldn't have been more fantastic. She's my biggest supporter and fan, and we have no secrets when it comes to my medical condition." Similarly, Jo Allen says that having a husband who makes her take good care of herself is her number one secret of living for 59 years with diabetes without any significant health problems. Jane Dohrmann also says that often her husband and son will notice that she's getting low before she does. "My best support person is my husband," she says. "He is tremendous and has saved my life from hypoglycemic episodes more times than I think any man should ever have to go through. My son is also a gem and has also saved me quite a few times himself."

Chuck Eichten has found additional benefits of involving a

supportive spouse. His wife has been very involved in his diabetes from the beginning of their courtship. "I'm so lucky. She has been tremendous," he says. "She digs into finding out the whys and the hows of what's going on with my diabetes." A major benefit, though, has been having both of them go to his doctor's appointments together. "We've found that two pairs of ears are better. We come home with so much more information between us when we both go." Also, after carrying the burden of diabetes alone for many of his 31 years with diabetes, he finds that it's nice to share it. His wife was involved in his decision to go on an insulin pump, which has taken away his bad lows and seizures and changed his life for the better. "Even my wife said how much of a positive effect the pump has had on me and on our relationship," Chuck remarks. "She said she doesn't worry about me all the time now. You don't always realize how taxing your diabetes can be to other people."

Similarly, Will Speer, Sr., credits his wife with being a tremendous support and a large part of the reason that he has lived so long with diabetes. "She provides me with three good meals a day. The only problem is that she's such a super cook that I have to fight my weight!" Rabbi Meisels says that his wife, Leah, also worries about him and makes sure that his portions are measured so that he can count carbs more easily. Likewise, Marc Blatstein says the best support person in his life is his wife Jill. "Not only is she my best friend, but she also looks after me, gives me hell when I deserve it, and helps me in any way that I need. She has had a head start when it comes to knowing about diabetes, since her older sister has been living with type 1 for the last 40 years."

The youngest child in a large family, Bernadette McIntyre says that her older brothers and sisters were very supportive, as well as her parents, while Anna Maria Gould credits much of her continued good health to the support of her family, husband, and son. Carol Sawyer advises all people with diabetes to get their spouses and families involved in their care. "My husband has gotten so involved in every aspect of my health," she acknowledges. For Julie Krupnick, having a supportive family is important not only for all of these reasons, but also because it gives her someone to vent to about her blood sugar control that really "gets it."

Even if you're not married or don't have a significant other in your life, it's still important to involve other people. Mary Sue Rubin recommends that it helps to have friends, family, and coworkers who are supportive. What's more, her older brother, Richard Rubin, PhD, is a clinical psychologist specializing in diabetes care even though he doesn't have the disease himself. A past-president of the American Diabetes Association, he has been involved in his sister's care at times, as well as in the care of his son, Stefan, who also has type 1 diabetes. Barbara Baxter, who also lives alone, has had some friends who will call to check on her, along with her sister, who calls her most mornings to make sure she's not too low. Similarly, Grant McArthur has a cousin in San Diego where he lives and friends who have been supportive, along with some past girlfriends. His roommate of more than ten years is probably the most supportive of all, though. "He has caught me having low blood sugars before I realized it," he says. "I think that sometimes it's scarier for him than for me."

Don Gifford agrees with all of them to a point, stating, "You can't do it without the support of family members and other partners, but there's a fine balance between concern and intervention." Sometimes, your family and friends mean well, but their support can be smothering. There's a fine line between their being supportive and overly concerned with your health. So, the key is to involve your family members and close friends in your diabetes care, but make sure they also know when to back off and stop hovering. Although Bill King credits his wife, a nurse, with teaching him a lot about diabetes after his diagnosis, he also sees the benefits of having such boundaries. He says, "My wife and I have come to an understanding about my lows. I rarely need help, but when I do, she just asks me to check my blood sugar instead of sticking some food in my face."

Others are unsure at times how to react to your diabetes. Dee Brehm says her friends try to be supportive when they're around her. "I have two close friends who have the opposite reaction when we go out to lunch. One makes excessive comments about the deliciousness of the desserts whenever we eat; the other one won't eat dessert when I'm around to be supportive." In either case, at least they're aware of her diabetes, although they have different ways of dealing with it. Just the fact that they acknowledge Dee's diabetes (even in their own, opposing ways) likely increases her overall happiness level by making her feel cared about by her friends.

Although Dr. Steve's two daughters tested negative for diabetes when they were young (and still have no signs of it as teenagers), he still considers his clan as one big happy diabetes family. Admittedly, his girls have lived their entire lives in an environment surrounded by diabetes-related products and information. "I can't tell you how many times I have dragged them to a diabetes conference that my wife and or I were attending or a TCOYD conference," he says. "At least they understand diabetes, and if nothing else, they'll know how to prevent themselves from ever getting type 2."

For Peter Gariti, he feels that involving his wife and two daughters in his diabetes care has improved their health as well. "Both of my daughters have taken a page out of my book growing up," he states. "Neither one has any sign of diabetes, but they both are very health conscious from eating the same healthy meals my wife cooked for me. They never even realized that other people eat sugary cereals for breakfast until they went over to someone else's house." When it comes right down to it, our family members may have benefited in myriad health-related ways, too, which is just another reason you can choose to look at your diabetes as a blessing of sorts, instead of a curse.

40

Share Your Diabetes with Others

Another common secret of diabetes longevity is to "come out of the closet" and share the fact that you have diabetes with others. So many old-timers hid their diabetes from others for years, Dr. Sheri included. "I had diabetes from before I ever started kindergarten, but I still have people I knew in high school and college that never had a clue that I have it." Stories like hers are not uncommon. Similarly, when Judy Tripathi was diagnosed in elementary school, she didn't tell anyone, nor did she want anyone to know. "I was mortified to have to go to the school nurse every morning." Barbara Baxter also hid her diabetes after she was diagnosed at the age of 12. "I didn't want to tell people that I had diabetes when I was in my teens because I didn't want to be different," she admits. Peter Gariti also found it easier to keep his diabetes hidden when he was younger. "I found out early on," he recounts, "that telling people I had diabetes was more trouble than it was worth—mainly for the other people. At birthday parties, my friends' mothers who knew used to fuss over me, so I rarely told anyone, although I still watched what I ate."

Mary Sue Rubin had a similar experience. "My biggest fear was that people would know I have diabetes." Now, though, she thinks that one of the secrets to living well with diabetes is to be open about having it instead of hiding it. Likewise, after hiding his diabetes through elementary and high school and even five years spent abroad in Israel afterward, S. Fasten finally came out of his "closet" and got some much-needed help.

"Someone found out I had diabetes and encouraged me to go to a diabetes meeting. It was only then that I found out that my knowledge level about diabetes was very low. I got a new doctor, read Dr. Bernstein's book, and got in much better control."

Nowadays, there is no reason to feel ashamed or embarrassed about having diabetes, and it's oftentimes a lot harder to hide, what with insulin pumps, continuous glucose monitors, and other visible reminders. Since there's not such a stigma attached to having it now, it's also a lot easier to share, plus most people know at least something about it given the current diabetes epidemic and all of the press it has gotten lately. Also, kids are learning more about diabetes than people in their age groups ever knew before. In fact, some kids even do show-and-tells at school with their insulin pumps.

Jim Turner says he wants other actors on the set to know that he has diabetes, but instead of bringing it up in conversation, he simply pulls out his blood glucose meter and tests in front of them. Sometimes, then, people will comment on his meter, and he talks to them about what's involved with having diabetes. He uses moments like those as teachable ones, viewing them as a chance to get rid of some of the ignorance that still exists about diabetes. For Chuck Eichten, his conversation starter is his insulin pump, but it serves the same purpose. "My pump has helped me become more public about my diabetes," he says. "I'm more comfortable talking about it. People see me pull out my pump, and they ask me questions."

Without a doubt, sharing your diabetes in certain settings has not always been the best practice. Long-timers with diabetes have often had to worry about discrimination in jobs due to diabetes, for good reason. For a long time, Judy Tripathi would apply for jobs and never tell anyone about her diabetes, although she is now mortified about having done so. She may have been insightful in not telling prospective employers, though. Will

Speer, Sr., was discharged from the Navy due to his diabetes diagnosis at the age of 27. He remembers applying for jobs afterward, only to be rejected as if he had a contagious disease whenever he admitted having diabetes. For a while, he was very worried about being able to find a job, any job. Although he went to work for the merchant marines and then the U.S. Postal Service, he still felt like people were making assumptions about his ability to work based on his diabetes alone. "They kept telling me that I wouldn't be able to do things alone (like going out on a postal route), and I kept proving them wrong."

Bob Cleveland also reminisces about his early experiences with discrimination in the workplace due to diabetes. "I majored in accounting, but then lost several jobs after admitting that I have diabetes." As noted in his profile earlier in this book, he finally stopped telling prospective employers that he had diabetes, and withholding that vital information about his health was the only way finally landed a good accounting job. Today, though, he's proud of his diabetes and freely shares his experiences. If he were trying to get a job nowadays, he would also be less likely to suffer from discrimination as a result of such a disclosure.

The American Diabetes Association in particular has worked long and hard to prevent diabetes-related work discrimination by establishing a national call center that handles requests for information and complaints in their Legal Advocacy office. Since most of the discrimination diabetic individuals experience is the result of decision makers' ignorance of diabetes and current management methods, the ADA first tries to educate, but then it is prepared to negotiate, litigate, and legislate as necessary to prevent or stop ongoing cases of discrimination. If you need their assistance in a job- or school-related diabetes matter, contact their main offices at 800-DIABETES.

Similarly, Marc Blatstein never hesitates to speak out about having diabetes or the issues he has had with living with it for close to 50 years, which is beneficial for everyone involved. "I've taught and counseled many tens of thousands—probably over 100,000—with diabetes over the past 20 years. The counseling, in a roundabout way, has been good medicine for me," he admits. Rabbi Meisels agrees. "By helping others, you gain a lot yourself," he contends. "You will get to practice what you preach. God will also reward you for your merit of doing good deeds." He should know, given that he has established the Friends with Diabetes organization that helps all Jewish people facing the challenge of diabetes and addresses culturally specific issues of heritage, lifestyle, and cuisine. Regardless of what personal rewards you get as compensation, the mere act of sharing your diabetes with others will likely benefit your own psyche equally in positive ways.

Another reason to share your diabetes with others is to help dispel other myths and ignorance about diabetes that still abound. "So few people understand about having a low blood sugar," says Freddi Fredrickson. "You can be having a low today, and three weeks later your friends might ask you how you're feeling."

Ron DeNunzio says, "One of my barriers was that I did not know any better. The way I was feeling, I thought I was fine." He first started having diabetic complications in the 1980s after less than 20 years with poorly controlled diabetes. "I still meet people who say, 'You never took care of yourself. This is why you are the way you are.' I look at them and then I try to explain to them about diabetes, to educate them. At the end of our conversation, I have changed their outlook on diabetes most of the time."

41

Find a Diabetes Hero or Mentor

Sometimes having someone else in your life who has had diabetes and who made a major impact on you—a friend, hero, or mentor—can make all the difference in the care you take of yourself. Marc Blatstein's "diabetic hero" was his aunt, whom he credits with saving his life. The two of them were very close, but she died from diabetic complications when he was 29 years old. He was with her in her nursing home near the end of her life, at which point she had lost her sight, her toes, and a foot, and she had other diabetes-related health problems as well. Not long before her death, she told him, "Marc, please don't do to yourself what I did to myself, and make a difference!" With those words, his own life with diabetes turned around, and he realized, "I couldn't divorce my diabetes or fire it, so I decided to make it my partner in life." He also had a friend and mentor in his first endocrinologist, Dr. Robert Kay. "Dr. Kay would take me with him on his daily rounds at the Children's Hospital of Philadelphia when I was diagnosed and staying there," Marc shares. "I was in the Children's Hospital for approximately six weeks. He encouraged me to laugh and smile with diabetes. He stayed a friend throughout my life. Dr. Kay was also one of the cofounders of the Juvenile Diabetes Research Foundation. He was my inspiration and my guiding light, and I was lucky to have him as my physician and friend."

For Ron DeNunzio, his niece is part of his support system and his chosen "hero." He already had diabetes when she was diagnosed with diabetes at the age of 5. He says of his niece, "She makes me want to become a better person with diabetes and live a long and healthy life. I need to show Emily that diabetes is okay." On the flip side, another hero of his is the endocrinologist he went to see in the 1990s, Dr. James Lenhard, who helped Ron turn his life with diabetes around once and for all. "He told me I could become a better person with diabetes," Ron recalls. "Those words meant so much to me; this doctor cared. I had eye problems and was missing half of my left foot at the time. He knew the road I was taking, and he changed my life."

Sometimes, it's just as beneficial to be someone else's hero, to give him (or her) another person to look up to or admire. Along those lines, Rich Humphreys tries to inspire kids with diabetes all the time at the summer camp for diabetic kids (Camp Ho Mita Koda) near Cleveland, Ohio, that he has been directing for the last twenty-plus years (see his profile for a good story about his latest exploits there). Paul McGuigan spends his summers working at the same camp as Rich. He says, "The people who I have met at camp over the years have been very influential in my life." He is also the director for a type 2 diabetic kids' camp that takes place there as well. In addition, Paul found himself another mentor and friend, a young doctor who hired Paul to work as a study coordinator for an NIH-funded study on type 2 diabetes in kids. This doctor, sadly, ended up recently dying from cancer, but Paul has a goal to carry on his legacy. "He taught me how to deal with families of kids with diabetes, professionals, and others. He was always there with the right answer. I plan to carry on his work."

Jane Dohrmann has been both on the receiving and giving end of being a diabetes hero or mentor. She says, "I was blessed with the help and friendship of a woman many years ago. The friendship took place when I was first diagnosed. She was also a juvenile diabetic and had been since the age of 8. She was my mentor before 'mentor' was a fashionable word." Jane's mentor taught her about what women have to go through with diabetes.

Unfortunately, this woman died at the age of 54 before heart stents and other lifesaving treatments were available. Jane herself recently had two stents placed in her coronary arteries to relieve blockage there, but she wishes that the treatment had been available sooner to help her mentor live a longer life.

Learning from her mentor that giving is always better than receiving, Jane says, "I have always tried to be that kind of person to others." In many cases, her support of other people with diabetes has made a difference. For instance, at one diabetes support group she was attending a number of years ago, she overheard a young diabetic boy's parents talking about him and how they felt responsible for their 4-year-old's condition. Jane recalls, "There were doing everything for the little boy, and the more I sat there and listened, the more I felt I had to say something." At a break in the session, she offered her help. "I told them it was vital that they begin to allow their son to take responsibility for some of the duties associated with diabetes. They said they felt it was their duty, and I explained to them that he was going to need all the knowledge he could when he grew up. He also was going to need to know that this wasn't anyone's fault . . . especially not the fault of his parents." She later heard from her nurse that a woman and her husband who had attended a support group had been talking about a lady who had given them some wonderful advice about caring for their diabetic son; the woman they were referring to was Jane, who says, "I was so relieved that these people were comfortable with the suggestions I had made. Their son must be a teenager by now, and I hope he's doing well." If using your own experiences like Jane and others have to help people besides yourself live better lives with diabetes doesn't make you feel good, then nothing will.

RICH HUMPHREYS, AGE 65, LIVING WITH TYPE 1

DIABETES 51 YEARS

What would make a normally mild-mannered, 14-year-old kid come home and kick a floor lamp across the room? A visit with his doctor, who told a newly diagnosed, ninth grader named Rich Humphreys that he couldn't wrestle on the varsity wrestling team for his school "for a while" because of his diabetes, of course. Although he eventually got to wrestle again, this was the first of many hurdles that Rich's condition has erected during his lifetime. Since that time, he has learned that a positive attitude can get you through about anything. "You have to view life as an adventure and have fun," he advises.

Rich is definitely in the habit of following his own advice and turning life's lemons into lemonade. He had been an art teacher, but when diabetes made him start to lose his eyesight and his vocation, he decided to set up a nature trail for children, along which they could look for gnomes and learn more about protecting nature and the environment. He had even put a rope guide along the trail so that he would be able to do it even when his sight was gone. Luckily for him, although he was blind in one eye for a year and a half, laser treatments for retinopathy and a vitrectomy served to restore his sight almost completely. He still guides kids through the nature trail, though, and inspires them with his courage and inspirational stories along the way.

Much to his credit, Rich has also been heavily involved with a camp for diabetic children and adolescents thirty miles east of Cleveland, Ohio, Camp Ho Mita Koda (which means "welcome, my friend" in Sioux), both as director for over two decades and "chief of inspiration." For instance, in September 2005, he walked 380 miles from the camp to his home in South Lancaster County, Pennsylvania, to both raise money for the camp and to make a statement to kids with diabetes. It took him five weeks wearing forty pounds of gear. He did have one bad low blood sugar reaction during the trip, when he woke up shaking and couldn't find his glucose tablets. "I flipped open my cell phone to call the friend I was meeting the next day, and using the light on my cell, I found my glucose tablets," he recalls.

He attributes his longevity with diabetes to a combination of secrets. After viewing life as an adventure, he also places having a sense of humor high on his list. "You have to have it with a chronic disease," he says. He also sees diabetes as a teacher, and he has learned to look at it philosophically. He monitors his blood glucose faithfully, but not compulsively; tries not to worry about the possibility of getting other diabetic complications; eats a healthy diet (he even makes his own bread with almond flour); continues to be a role model, especially for diabetic kids; cultivates a grateful heart; exercises regularly; and works doing things he loves. A final secret he swears by is an herbal supplement called quercetin, recommended to him by Dr. Eugene Shippen, which has completely cured the neuropathy he was developing in his legs.

Most of all, Rich simply never lets life get him down for long. He had a goal to go around the world by the time he reached 33 years of age, and he accomplished it all without a blood glucose meter and even with a few bad low blood sugars. He still kept on going—and we're certain that he'll be leading the rest of us on adventures for many more years to come!

PART EIGHT

Other Life Secrets

42

Have Kids If You Want To

Many women with diabetes in the not-so-distant past were counseled not to have children. However, a lot of them did anyway, with great success due to their vigilant control over their diabetes. Marcy Shefsky is one such example. "I lost two children," she recalls, "but my endocrinologist said it wasn't due to diabetes." Between natural births and adoptions, she ended up with three healthy children anyway. The limit for Gladys Dull was one child, born back in 1947. "I never thought I would have kids at all," she says. "No one told me not to have any, but they did tell me that I wouldn't be able to have any more after I had to have a C-section for my son Norm to be born."

Another example is Patty Schaeffer, who was told that she wouldn't be able to have children because of her diabetes. She and her fiancé were both Catholic, so they talked about the possibility of adoption after her doctor's devastating pronouncement before their marriage. What happened instead, though, was that after they married, she bore five healthy children in six years. "It's the only way to do it," she remarks, implying that if you're going to have that many kids, whether or not you have diabetes, you might as well get all the pregnancies over with in as few years as possible. Enter into the picture again the Joslin Diabetes Center (then called the Joslin Clinic). "My husband was in the Navy, and we were stationed in Newport, Rhode Island. The Navy doctor sent me to the Joslin Clinic, and I was in the hospital for most of my first pregnancy and during parts of two of the others." She feels that she was fortunate to deal with informed doctors throughout her pregnancies and learn various ways to control her diabetes better. "Being at the Joslin for the first one really helped me to know what to do for the rest of them," she says, happily reporting that all five of her babies did well.

Anna Maria Gould got engaged in college, and both she and her fiancé wanted to have children badly; she had been raised in a family of six, while he was one of seven kids in his family. However, her gynecologist told her that she should not have any children, warning her that her life could be in jeopardy because her diabetes would cause her body to go through too much stress during pregnancy (which she had been diagnosed with at the age of 9). Although her fiancé was wonderful about it and completely understanding, Anna decided to research it for herself and subsequently started seeing an endocrinologist, one who told her that it was possible for her to have a child. Two years later, she became pregnant and had a healthy baby boy. "It took proper care and consistent blood glucose monitoring," she remembers. "I had to go to the hospital frequently back then for blood draws, since meters weren't widely available then yet." She attributes getting through it to keeping on top of her blood sugars, reading up on pregnancies in diabetic mothers, and continuing to learn new things that helped with her control.

Luckily for Carolyn Balcom, she was able to go through her

first pregnancy without having to worry about diabetes, since she was not diagnosed until she was 28 years old (in 1964) and was breast-feeding her first child. With the support of her husband, she had two more after her diagnosis, but the last one looked more like a baby of a diabetic mother, weighing over nine pounds (although the first two were closer to seven). After her third, her obstetrician suggested that she not have any more children, and she took his advice.

HOW DO YOU KNOW IF YOU HAVE GESTATIONAL DIABETES?

This type of diabetes is usually diagnosed when you've reached twenty-four to twenty-eight weeks of pregnancy, at which point most obstetricians will have you do a screening test. You'll likely be asked to drink Glucola, which contains fifty grams of glucose, and they'll check your blood sugar levels one hour later. If your value is at or above 140 mg/dl at one hour, you'll either be diagnosed with gestational diabetes or be asked to do a three-hour oral glucose tolerance test (involving 100 grams of glucose) on another day. If you do the second test, your blood glucose should be below 180 mg/dl after one hour, 155 at two hours, and 140 at the end to be considered normal. If you can't stomach straight glucose, your physician may simply have you eat eighteen Brach & Brock (or other type of) jelly beans as an alternative test.

Some physicians advocate only screening women with risk factors for diabetes, but doing so would likely miss about half of women with the gestational type. If you have a lot of risk factors for it (e.g., obese, glucose intolerant, prior history of gestational diabetes, family history of type 2, previous baby weighing over nine pounds), you should likely be screened early in pregnancy and again at twenty-four to twenty-eight weeks, if the early screening is negative. If you do experience gestational diabetes, be vigilant for signs of symptoms of type 2 diabetes afterward as having it during pregnancy greatly increases your risk for developing type 2 later on.

Nowadays, a diabetic woman (with type 1, type 2, or gestational) can easily have a successful pregnancy without fear of harming herself or causing birth defects in her child. No physician should be advising diabetic women not to have children, unless she has severe health complications that would be worsened by a pregnancy or completely uncontrolled blood glucose levels. When it comes to diabetic mothers having successful pregnancies, blood glucose meters have been a godsend. Dr. Sheri remembers thinking that she would never be able to have any kids, particularly since she was having some problems with unstable proliferative diabetic retinopathy in her mid-20s (when she had already had diabetes for over two decades). She waited until her eyes had fully stabilized following laser treatments (which took about two years) before she even considered the possibility of going through a pregnancy.

"I researched all I could about diabetes and pregnancy," Dr. Sheri says. "I looked up the possibility of a pregnancy making my eyes unstable again. I also wanted to know how much of a chance I had of passing diabetes on to my kids. I had to feel like I was doing everything I could to prevent my babies from getting birth defects by normalizing my blood sugars before I even got pregnant." She entered into a prepregnancy study looking at the effects of normalizing blood sugars on pregnancy outcomes, mainly to gain further tools to help her prevent problems, and then she took the plunge and got pregnant on her first try.

The ease of her pregnancy really surprised her. "When I tried to keep my blood sugars from ever going over 120 even an hour after eating before I was pregnant, it was hard work, and I wasn't always successful. I was testing every hour practically all day long, and I wondered if I'd ever be able to do it when I was actually pregnant. But when I was carrying my son, controlling my blood sugars was actually easier. Sure, your insulin needs go up during the pregnancy, but it's gradually changing, which is not at all like dealing with my normal monthly hormonal swings. My blood sugars have never been more stable and manageable than during my three, successful pregnancies. Any problems I had with my pregnancies were not related at all to my diabetes."

Dr. Sheri had one C-section (not because of diabetes, but rather because of a heart-shaped uterus that made her son stay sideways), followed by two vaginal deliveries, all without a single problem with her eye health or diabetes. Her three terrific (and so far non-diabetic) sons are currently 13, 11, and 8 years old. "Definitely get yourself in good control first," she advises anyone who is contemplating having kids, "and then go for it."

Bernadette McIntyre, who has two children, agrees. "Get yourself under control and get a good obstetrician," she advises. She also recommends using an insulin pump, if you have that option. "It's the best route to take," she says. Dr. Sheri went through her first two pregnancies using the now off-the-market Ultralente basal insulin, but she used an insulin pump during her last one. She is of the same mind as Bernadette when it comes to pump use during pregnancy. "It's not that you can't make other insulin regimens work for you. I did just fine not using one the first two times. It's just much easier to keep adjusting your basal doses up during your pregnancy—which you will invariably have to do—when you're using an insulin pump." Even women experiencing gestational diabetes (which occurs primarily in the third trimester when anti-insulin hormones are raging) can benefit from going on an insulin pump for the remainder of their pregnancies.

Karen Poenisch agrees that good control during your pregnancies is critical and that it can be done. "You wish you could be in that good of control all the time," she admits. Karen's story about having two sons (now ages 23 and 22) is an inspiration. When she was diagnosed with some retinopathy at the age of 21, just six months after she was married, the doctor told her that she

SURE-FIRE PREGNANCY TIPS FOR WOMEN WITH PREEXISTING OR GESTATIONAL DIABETES

- For the best pregnancy outcomes, keep blood sugars in nondiabetic ranges at all times (< 100 mg/dl), and avoid glucose spikes (>120 mg/dl) one to two hours after eating.
- If you were taking oral medications prior to getting pregnant, your doctor will likely put you on insulin during your pregnancy (basal + bolus regimen) because the safety of most diabetes medications for your baby is not known.
- Going on insulin during the last part of your pregnancy can help keep your blood sugars under control, if you can't do it through dietary and other means.
- Watch your carbohydrate intake carefully (by counting carbs), and restrict your intake of refined (rapidly absorbed) carbs at all times.
- Eat smaller meals or become a grazer during your pregnancy.
- Exercise fifteen to sixty minutes daily throughout your pregnancy to lower blood glucose levels and prevent excess weight gain, fatigue, and often gestational diabetes.
- If you have type 2 or gestational diabetes and didn't use insulin before pregnancy, exercising regularly may prevent your going on it or allow you to take smaller doses.
- Switch to non-weight-bearing workouts (like stationary cycling or water exercise) later in your pregnancy, and avoid exercises done lying flat on your back.
- Limit your workout to an easy or moderate intensity, but avoid vigorous workouts (like heavy weight training).
- Avoid exercise in the heat and excessively prolonged bouts of activity (more than an hour) done without a break.
- Monitor your blood sugars before, during, and after exercise, and eat additional carbohydrate snacks as needed to prevent low blood sugars.
- If you have high blood pressure, preterm labor, placenta previa, heart or lung disease, or a baby that is not growing well, consult your physician before starting exercise.

wouldn't be able to have kids and advised her to get sterilized. Luckily, she decided to wait. She got a blood glucose meter in 1980 and then went on an insulin pump, finally using the combination to get into better control. She was in her late 20s when she had both of her sons. "I was in perfect control when I was pregnant, and they were perfect when they were born. I was the first diabetic mother where I lived in Texas to have normal babies, so everyone came to see them," she recalls. To date, her vision loss from retinopathy has been minimal, even with her pregnancies. "They're so great," she says of her sons. "I love them."

On the other hand, most diabetic men have not been advised against having children because of their disease. Jim Arthur says that he had even talked to some medical people who told him not to worry about having diabetic offspring. (Incidentally, the chances of having a diabetic child are lower for diabetic mothers—about 2 percent—than for diabetic men, who have closer to a 6 percent chance.) He now has two sons in their 40s with no sign of diabetes, along with four, healthy, nondiabetic grandchildren. Interestingly, Rabbi Meisels was advised against having four or more children. The rationale behind stopping at three had nothing to do with diabetes, though. He recalls, "The doctors told me that when I got married, I shouldn't have more than three kids because I need to have a stress-free life." When he and his wife had their fourth one, he said to himself, "The doctor's wrong. Thank you, God." He now has five kids . . . and possibly more coming. His story makes Dr. Sheri and Dr. Steve want to know what his doctors were thinking because for him to have a stress-free life, they probably should have advised him never to have any kids!

43

Always Expect the Unexpected When You Travel

Always expect the unexpected" should be the diabetic motto for traveling or being away from home for an extended period. Although you can't avoid the occasional surprise, preparation before you leave on a trip or long outing can help you avoid undue stress. For instance, you should come prepared with extra supplies, medications, and even extra batteries for your glucose meter (and insulin pump, if you wear one). Some countries require you to have written documents from your doctor stating that you're allowed to carry medicines or supplies, particularly syringes and needles. It's also helpful to bring copies of all of your prescriptions and a list of your medications, including how much you take of each and when (even your doses of different insulins).

Furthermore, you will want to carry all of your diabetes-related supplies with you on board the plane (or at least half of them), if that's the way you're traveling. Placing them in checked baggage that could potentially be lost or delayed is asking for trouble (particularly nowadays with all of the heightened travel security measures and large number of checked bags). If you are going abroad for a long period of time, you may want to send your additional supplies via insured or trackable mail to your destination prior to leaving. Insulin is best to keep with you in the climate-controlled airplane cabin, since checked baggage is exposed to greater ranges of temperatures than your carry-on items.

Other problems can arise if you have to buy supplies or insulin outside of the United States. American-sold insulins are all U-100 strength, but other countries may sell more dilute U-40 or U-80 varieties, which require different syringes to match these insulins. If you use the wrong syringe, you can make a mistake in your insulin dose such as taking too little insulin when using U-100 syringes with lower-strength insulins. If you travel to certain areas of the world, diabetic supplies may be even harder to come by or expensive to get without your usual insurance coverage.

The American Diabetes Association also recommends that you start your trip with at least double the supplies that you think you'll need during your trip, carry a quick-acting source of glucose to treat hypoglycemia in-flight, and bring a snack like a nutrition bar that travels well. The ADA additionally suggests that you carry or wear medical identification and bring your physician's contact information with you. If feasible, you may also want to have a list of potential health-care professionals at your destination, especially English-speaking ones if you're not fluent in the languages of the countries you're visiting. Finally, be prepared to adjust your timing of medications appropriately when traveling to different time zones. For shorter travel within the United States, though, Dr. Sheri finds it easiest to simply leave her watch on its usual Eastern time and give all long-acting insulins on the same schedule that she normally follows, and others, like Rabbi Meisels, choose to do the same when the time change is three or fewer hours.

One example of a diabetic traveler is Jim Arthur. When he was still working (before his retirement), he lived in Belgium for three years and always got his supplies in the United States, so he didn't have to buy insulin or testing supplies in Europe. He traveled all over the world for his job, though, and he avoided problems by always keeping the supplies he needed with him. Likewise, to assist with his glucose control when he travels longer distances, Rabbi Meisels also wears the DexCom continuous glucose monitor. "It's not the most accurate tool," he admits, "but it comes in handy, especially when I travel nowadays."

No matter how well you plan ahead, it's hard to cover every possible contingency. For instance, S. Fasten from Brooklyn, New York, once journeyed to Israel with a limited number of infusion sets for his pump. Unfortunately for him, he had inserted his last set incorrectly, but he didn't realize it until his blood sugars climbed to 400. He had thirty-six hours before he would be back to the United States, and he was luckily able to "borrow" a syringe from someone and had enough insulin (albeit short-acting) to get him home without going into diabetic ketoacidosis. Had he followed the diabetic travelers' motto, he would have brought along extra infusion sets, along with a spare syringe or two.

DIABETES TRAVEL TIPS FROM THE U.S. TRANSPORTATION SECURITY ADMINISTRATION (TSA)

- When going through the initial TSA screening process, let the screeners know that you have diabetes and will be carrying your supplies with you.
- Clearly identify your insulin and insulin dispensers (e.g., vials, jet injectors, pens, infusers, and preloaded syringes) with a prescription label with your name on it.
- Your other liquid prescription medicines, such as Symlin, Byetta, and glucagon, must also be clearly identified with a prescription label that matches your ID.
- If you have liquids and gels (including cake icing) to treat hypoglycemia in larger than three-ounce containers, you must declare these items to security checkpoint personnel.
- You may carry on an unlimited number of unused syringes as long as you also have vials of insulin or other injectable medications with you (although used syringes must be in a sharps disposal or another approved container) .

- In addition, you may carry on blood glucose meters and test strips, continuous blood glucose monitors, lancets, alcohol swabs, control solutions, and other blood glucose-monitoring supplies.
- You are free to wear your insulin pump (but advise the screeners that you are wearing it) and carry on all of your insulin pump supplies.
- If you would rather have all of your diabetes-related supplies inspected visually rather than have them go through x-ray inspection, you will need to package all of them in a separate bag to be handed to the screeners before you pass through the checkpoint.
- As travel and security guidelines are constantly in a state of flux, check with a travel agent, TSA (866-289-9673), or the American Diabetes Association (800-DIABETES or www.diabetes.org) to make sure that no new requirements have come into effect that will impact your travel with diabetes supplies.

During your travels, you should also expect that your blood sugars may not respond the way they normally do and will likely be more variable than usual. Dr. Steve finds that traveling is particularly hard because he's eating different foods and varying the timing of his meals. "It probably the most difficult situation I have to deal with," he says. He travels frequently, attending professional meetings, giving lectures, and putting on TCOYD conferences all over the country, so he has first-hand experience dealing with the additional challenges that traveling with diabetes entails.

Likewise, Bill King travels for the insulin pump company that he works for (and to teach people about exercise at TCOYD cConferences), and he experiences similar challenges. "My body is certainly sensitive to the stress of travel," he says. "I usually need more insulin." The biggest factor for him that affects his blood sugars is sitting for long periods of time. The inactivity in airports, on planes, or in his car causes his blood sugars to rise, and he has to work to stay in control by increasing his basal rate on his insulin pump and monitoring more frequently. A good antidote to these travel difficulties is to try to move around whenever you can. Get up and walk up and down the aisle on the airplane periodically or at least stand up next to your assigned seat, walk around in the airport when you're waiting for your flight to depart, and sit as little as possible whenever you're not forced to during your trip. Dr. Sheri particularly dislikes long car trips because she finds that the long stretches of inactivity (which are unusual for her) always makes her blood sugars go up. "I eat less and give more insulin but still have a hard time keeping my blood sugars under control during long trips," she complains.

For others, the stress involved in traveling alone can cause a rise in glucose levels. For instance, Matthew Lore experiences increases in his blood sugars when he flies—partly, he believes, from being more sedentary for longer stretches of time than he usually is, but also because he's somewhat stressed by not being in control of his mode of transportation (in his day-to-day life, he gets nearly everywhere he goes by bicycle). "If I were the one flying the plane, I would probably be okay," he says. Even the stress of running late to make a connecting flight (or missing one) or hitting unexpected traffic on the way to the airport can cause your blood sugars to rise, along with the additional frustrations associated with check-in and other delays associated with current security-tight conditions.

Along the same lines, the physical stress of traveling—including lack of sleep, time zone changes, altered eating patterns and timing, and more—can contribute to increases in cortisol as well, which will only serve to make your insulin work less well and cause your doses to rise. You will likely need to plan ahead and bring as many of your own snacks with you as you can to prevent or treat hypoglycemia and to have a modicum of control over the foods that you have access to during your trip. Also, you should never assume that you will have access to food wherever you go, particularly in unfamiliar or foreign places. All in all, you will need to be more vigilant about monitoring your diabetes control and preventing potential problems from multiple sources whenever you're traveling.

❧ 44 ❧

Do What You Like to Do

Pursuing activities that have nothing to do with diabetes can help get your focus off of it twenty-four hours a day, seven days a week. For example, if you find a sense of purpose in your job, focus more on it. Enjoying your work situation makes it easier to deal with the inevitable diabetes- or just life-related setback when it comes along. As Rich Humphreys advises, "Find work that you love." Both Dr. Steve and Dr. Sheri find gratification in working hard to help others deal more effectively with their diabetes by organizing diabetes conferences, conducting research studies, and writing books and articles on the topic.

If your work doesn't divert your focus enough, look for enjoyment in your hobbies, activities, community organizations, or religious participation. Mary Sue Rubin fervently believes that part of her long-term success with diabetes has come from having outside interests—friends, hobbies, etc.—to focus on. "They help keep your mind off of diabetes," she asserts. Studies have even shown that older individuals participating in regular social dancing have enhanced gait and balance, so there may be physical health benefits to having outside interests in addition to psychological ones.

For Marc Blatstein, earning a first-degree black belt in Taek Won Do has been important in his life for both physical and mental reasons. He started practicing this martial art as a kid and has continued throughout his lifetime. He calls it "mind, body, and spirit medicine," and for him it has been very healing and motivational. In November of 2000, he competed in an international tournament in Mar del Plata, Argentina, where he won a third-place trophy in forms despite having had diabetes for four decades and being 50 years old at the time. He lost his chance at third place in sparring, though, due to an unexpected and ill-timed hypoglycemic reaction, but he still considers himself a winner because he had beaten diabetes again by even making it into the tournament. He coined a saying well before that event when he was interviewed for a story about his life with diabetes: "I am not just living with diabetes; I am winning with my diabetes." As it has done for Marc, finding outside interests and excelling in them despite diabetes can certainly help anyone win with diabetes.

Gerald Cleveland is another great example of someone who has had a multitude of outside interests to keep his focus diverted elsewhere. In addition to his many civic-minded activities, like being involved with and volunteering his time for a local PBS TV station, Junior Achievement, the Syracuse Rescue Mission, his local Presbyterian church, and his community at large, he spent ten years working on completing a doctoral degree in education (which he accomplished in 1961), while concurrently working full-time as the assistant superintendent of Syracuse's public school system. In fact, after 75 years with diabetes, he still keeps busy doing other things. He's active as the chairman of one of the committees in his retirement community, and he also volunteers his time to help others with diabetes learn how to eat correctly to better control their disease.

Many other diabetic individuals also keep busy, including Jane Dohrmann. She says, "Staying busy keeps you from dwelling on things that may otherwise worry you. There are simply some things that you can't do anything about—such as an unexplained high—so you keep busy, go, and do whatever you can to prevent it from happening again." Now that's advice that all of us can live with!

Finally, Dr. Steve advises that you take a commonsense approach to making any changes in your lifestyle to improve your diabetes control while doing what you want to do. "You have to do what works best for you," he says. For example, if you have to make dietary changes, he suggests that you come up with an individualized dietary program—one that is reflective of your culture or background—rather than one that works better for someone else. Also, pick the types of physical activities that are most enjoyable to you. Dr. Steve himself is currently more of a weekend warrior when it comes to exercise because his weekdays are so packed with work obligations. Nevertheless, he finds time to walk the dog, take bike rides, get in some pickup basketball games, and use his stepper, because those activities fit best into his lifestyle.

❧ 45 ❧

Adopt a Pet (or Two)

Not only are pets good for your mental health, but they can also teach you ways to better deal with having diabetes yourself. For Mary Sue Rubin, who has had diabetes almost half a century, animals have always been a big part of her life. Most of the cats and dogs she currently owns have medical problems themselves, and she thinks that their poor health has taught her to be more patient with herself. "Being aware of subtle changes in my animals' behavior has helped me learn to see those changes in myself. They've taught me patience and not to expect to have instant results." She also remarked that her pets help her keep a regular routine, which makes caring for her own diabetes easier.

For Gladys Dull, it has been a variety of pets that have kept her life more structured. "I have always loved animals," she recalls. She believes that pets help, much as Mary Sue Rubin does, by giving you something to focus on besides your own problems." My Schipperke is only 6 years old, but he has had kneecap problems," she says. During her previous 13 years of living in a home in the mountains, her family also had horses, which is how she had the opportunity to stay active by doing a lot of horseback riding.

Interestingly, a recent study investigated the fitness of dog walkers versus people who work out at a gym. The study was funded by a dog food company, but researchers still found that walking a dog daily lowered the owners' blood pressure, slowed their heart rates, reduced stress, and resulted in a quicker recovery from a burst of strenuous activity. Of the 1,500 people studied, the average dog walker covered a distance of 676 miles a year, which was over 200 miles more than gym goers got in. More importantly, most dog owners continued with their daily walking routine, whereas more than half of gym goers dropped out of their programs after two or three months. So, owning a dog that has to be walked, no matter what the weather is like, is one definite way to keep you more active and healthy.

Another positive benefit for dog owners is that having to walk their pet regularly increases social contact, which for many people enhances their feelings of happiness and social connectedness. Pets can be a conversation starter that leads to greater social interactions. As for other mental health benefits, studies have shown that interactions with pets can lower anxiety (who doesn't feel better after a tail-wagging welcome from your loving dog?)

and reduce stress. For people with diabetes, stress reduction is doubly important because it can also benefit blood sugar control. For cat lovers, sitting with a purring cat on your lap may be enough to change your outlook from negative to positive. Even watching tropical fish swim in a tank can bring about a sense of relaxation. If nothing else, having a pet to care for helps take your focus off of yourself and your own health for at least a few minutes a day. Whatever type of pet works best to alleviate your stress and improve your health should be the one you get.

❧ 46 ❧

Always Listen to Your Body

Interestingly, people who developed diabetes in the pre-meter era generally seem to have a greater awareness of changes in their blood glucose levels and other things. Perhaps it is a result of not having measurable means of knowing what their blood sugars were doing for many years and having to pay attention to changes in how they felt instead. Subtle changes and symptoms in your body are there, if you only take the time to look out for and listen to them.

For example, Dr. Sheri "knows" the glycemic effect of most foods without using a blood glucose meter. As a child, she knew which ones made her feel crappy (usually the ones that made her blood sugars rise rapidly), and to this day, she still steers clear of foods that "just aren't worth it" because of their potential and immediate impact on her energy levels, insulin needs, and more. "To this day, I still hardly need a glucose meter to tell me the glycemic effects of the foods I eat," she says. "Going for the first almost 20 years with diabetes without a meter gave me instantaneous feedback about their effects." She also chooses to avoid caffeine so that she can remain acutely aware of the initial symptoms of hypoglycemia. "When I start to feel the effects of adrenaline release like shakiness or a racing heart beat, I know it's from getting low and not a caffeine-induced effect." Others who are more habituated to the effects of caffeine or who are less sensitive to it than she is may not benefit as much from avoiding it, though.

Jim Turner also credits being focused on the way he felt before he had a blood glucose meter for his knowledge now of the effect foods have on him. "I was lucky to come into diabetes pretesting because I have a greater awareness of what's going on with my body," he comments. In agreement with him is Natalie Saunders, who says that one longevity secret is "to take notice of what's going on with your body." Actually, many of the people with diabetes before home glucose monitoring became available are very tuned in to how they feel when their blood sugars are high or low. Chuck Eichten also states that he has a really good sense of where his blood sugars are just from paying attention to his body. It's still hard to tell exactly where your blood glucose is when it's between about 80 and 180, though, as symptoms are generally not present until you get lower or higher than those levels, respectively.

Finally, if you look out for symptoms or slight changes in your body, you'll likely be able to pick up some conditions that can be treated or prevented before they become real issues. For instance, when Robert Mandell was walking in Florida with his lady friend a couple of years ago, he felt like he had bad indigestion. "It turns out," he recounts, "that I had angina and didn't even know it." After seeing a cardiologist, he ended up having a triple bypass, which corrected his coronary artery blockage *before* he ever suffered from a heart attack. Similarly, Zach Barneis recommends listening to your body and taking care of things as they arise. "Don't put things off, and don't go into denial," he advises. If you're tuned in, you may also pick up signs of infections or illness early on, as any type of physical stressor that requires your immune system to respond to it can also cause a rise in your blood sugar level. You can also pick up on when you're overly tired or emotionally stressed out as well. Marcy Shefsky says, "Get to know your body so you can fine-tune when something is going screwy. You can't wait to act." So, the best advice is probably to test your blood sugar whenever you have any doubts about how you feel and have other symptoms checked out by a doctor—and make it sooner rather than later.

47

Expect Your Body to Change

Aging is complex and causes its own set of bodily changes, many of which have nothing at all to do with diabetes. The aging process generally involves a gradual decline in the physiological function of your body's systems. Human cells apparently have a limited number of times that they can split and reproduce before dying, and once cells slow their rate of turnover, aging accelerates. The onset of some chronic diseases is often inseparable from aging, but many are not inevitable with advancing age. However, even if we could find a way to prevent all diseases from occurring, hospitals would still be full of people dying of nothing in particular except old age.

Prevention of an early death or impairment from preventable or treatable problems, though, is an essential part of longevity with and without diabetes. For example, your muscles start to lose more of their fibers that are not being routinely used with each passing decade, but being more physically active can offset such declines (at least to a point) and allow you to retain more of your muscular strength. The diabetes-related benefit is that having more insulin-sensitive muscle mass where glucose can be stored helps to keep your blood sugars under better control. Thus, to live long and well, you have to be vigilant about all aspects of your health, just like your nondiabetic friends need to be. With that goal in mind, seek out all the necessary doctors and specialists that you need to in order to stay healthy. As Larry Verity says, "Never assume that your health will be static. You have to get things treated and see all the necessary physicians—like a cardiologist, an ophthalmologist, and more." You should also address your mental health as well, since the stress of diabetes and life in general can affect your care.

One area of change related specifically to diabetes that can be quite challenging, though, is the fact that your symptoms of hypoglycemia may vary over time. What used to be your usual symptoms of getting low may no longer be the ones you get later on. What's more, your ability to sense low blood sugars may not stay constant either. Jo Allen's husband confirms just that. "Sometimes Jo's lows slip up on her now, and she doesn't realize it," he confides. "They didn't used to. If I can't get her to drink orange juice, I give her cake icing." Similarly, Jane Dohrmann frequently is no longer able to tell when she's getting low and to treat it in time, even though up until 2005 she had never had many bad lows at all. For Jim Arthur, his awareness has changed as well; he sensed his lows for most of his first six decades with diabetes, but in the last few years, he has developed some level of unawareness. "Nowadays I have to be careful about getting too low without knowing it," he says.

In addition to changes over time, you also need to pay attention to monthly, weekly, and daily changes in your insulin action, hormones, and more. For instance, in addition to the insulin-sensitizing effects of exercise, in premenopausal women the time of the month can affect how well their insulin works. Hormones like estrogen and progesterone released during the second half of the menstrual cycle (the luteal phase) can decrease the effects of insulin. In fact, many women experience dramatic differences in their insulin needs from the beginning on their monthly cycle to the end. "Estrogen makes your body less sensitive to insulin," says Dr. Sheri. Personally, she can often tell when her period is about to begin because all of a sudden, her blood sugars start dropping and keep on doing so for about the first twelve- to twenty-four hours, mainly due to the lowering of estrogen that occurs at that time. "The time of the month makes a huge difference to my insulin needs," she confirms, as can many other factors. As for men, loss of muscle mass and declining levels of testosterone can combine to reduce insulin action in their muscles as well. So, it's best to assume that care of your body and your diabetes will need to adapt over time to compensate for all such changes.

48

Never Start Smoking (or Stop Now)

As far as your health is concerned, smoking is one of the worst habits that you can adopt, and when you have diabetes, its effects on your health can be even more dramatic. In general, smokers are insulin resistant, exhibit several aspects of the insulin resistance syndrome, and have about a 50 percent higher risk of developing type 2 diabetes. If you have type 1 already, you may develop "double diabetes," or symptoms of both, from smoking. Moreover, smoking increases your risk of health complications from both microvascular (e.g., kidney, eye, and nerve problems) and macrovascular origins (heart attack, stroke, and peripheral vascular disease), probably via its metabolic effects in combination with increased inflammation around your body. The risk for microvascular problems is greatest in people with type 1 diabetes, while anyone with type 2 is more likely to develop heart disease or other cardiovascular problems. Thus, smoking cessation is of utmost importance to facilitate control over your blood sugars and to limit the possible development of diabetic complications.

Nicotine in tobacco causes the blood flow to your hands and feet to be severely restricted. Since those are the two primary areas of the body most commonly and negatively impacted by nerve damage caused by diabetes, adding smoking to the mix only exacerbates the potentially devastating effects on your feet and hands. As for heart and other blood flow problems, smoking is a major, independent risk factor for all types of cardiovascular problems in people without diabetes, and since diabetes itself is another strong risk factor, you're likely more than doubling your risk of having such problems if you smoke. As Bernadette McIntyre reminds us, "I do know from a cardiovascular standpoint that smoking constricts the blood vessels and for a diabetic this would further compromise a cardiovascular system that is at risk and especially needs extra care."

Dr. Sheri remembers meeting with her endocrinologist when she was a teenager and his telling her, "If you smoke, you'll die." His implication was that she would die sooner than expected from just having diabetes, and his message came through loud and clear.

She really hates being around cigarette smoke anyway, so not taking up smoking wasn't hard for her. Similarly, neither Gladys Dull, nor Dee Brehm, nor Carol Sessions, nor Barbara Baxter has ever smoked at all (except for Barbara's couple of weeks as a teen). Barbara does remember reading a lot about how bad it is for people with diabetes since that time, though. Likewise, Marc Blatstein also has never taken up the habit. "I received advice from my endocrinologist back in the 1980s about the negative effects of smoking in a support group meeting he ran." Grant McArthur listed one of his secrets of longevity with diabetes as being that he has never drunk alcohol or smoked cigarettes. (We agree with the no cigarettes part, but there may be some health benefits available to people with diabetes from moderate alcohol consumption, although Gladys Dull, the longest-living person with diabetes, also states that she has never drunk alcohol.)

Actually, none of the very longest-living diabetic individuals interviewed for this book smokes at present, although some of them did dabble with it for a while before its negative impact on health was fully understood. Al Lewis says, "I do not smoke now, although I did for about ten years during the period from 1961 to 1971. During that time, and subsequently, I did not receive medical advice relating to diabetes and smoking, but I do feel that if I were now smoking my endocrinologist would tell me to stop or find another physician!" Will Speer, Sr., also stopped smoking in 1971. "I was a smoker until cigarettes hit thirty-seven cents a pack; then they were too expensive. I only smoked about ten packs a week, but I took the three dollars and seventy cents a week I had been spending and saved it until I had enough to buy a suit. Back then, it didn't take long." A Vietnam veteran, he also says that back in the 1950s, the military used to provide them with cigarettes, going as far as to pack them in survival packs along with waterproof matches. "They don't do that anymore!" he adds.

While Patricia La France-Wolf did not smoke much more

than a pack a week, she did smoke from the time she was 18 until she went blind at 34. "I quit then—over 30 years ago," she recalls. "The doctors did tell me not to smoke." Freddi Fredrickson doesn't smoke now either, although she did smoke from about age 15 to when she turned 30. "I did receive some medical advice not to smoke," she says, "However, it was never emphatic. I stopped smoking because I couldn't stand the smell and worried about my lungs, not the effect on my diabetes." Jim Arthur smoked a pipe for a few years a long time ago, but he stopped—mainly because of its bad taste—and he never smoked cigarettes. Rabbi Meisels smoked, but just decided to stop on his own. The only person that ever gave him a hard time about it, though, was his wife.

Peter Gariti started smoking in college and continued to do so for about five years afterward. Luckily for him, he had a doctor at the time who advised him to stop (even though all of the negative effects of smoking were not well known at the time). Bob Elder stopped smoking for other reasons. "I was a smoker from college days (graduated in 1960) until 1997 when I retired. I had attempted to stop prior to that, and it was easy. I did it a bunch of times. The day I retired was the last time I smoked, and I think I was able to do it because the pressures of the job had been removed. My doctors, of course, used to tell me to stop, and certainly I knew that it was foolish, but I was addicted." Bob's reasoning gives us all just one more reason to try to control stress well through other means than smoking.

Don Gifford tells of an event that made him stop dabbling with cigarettes when he was young. "As a preteen and an early teen, I experimented with a few cigarettes as most boys in the early 1960s did. Then our 4-H club had a guest speaker that presented a color movie showing the lung surgery of a cancer victim. One guy in the club watching the movie passed out. Right after that, I quit experimenting with cigarettes." He admits to having smoked a pipe about five times a week during law school and for several years afterward, which he says seemed to provide him some physical comfort when his blood sugars were not as well controlled. "As my blood sugars became better controlled and the dangers of all forms of smoking became better known, I quit," he says. Mary Sue Rubin also admits to smoking for about a year during her rebellious period as a teenager.

Karen Poenisch reminds us again of what we all need to keep in mind: "Smoking is strongly related to circulation problems and heart disease. If I weren't a diabetes educator, my doc probably would have warned me about these risks. Smoking is not good." It's especially life-shortening for anyone with diabetes, so if you want to be a long-term diabetes survivor, right now is the time to stop smoking if you haven't already.

❦ 49 ❧

Keep Mentally Active

If you have prediabetes or any type of diabetes, you run a much higher risk of experiencing mental declines, often related to plaque formation in the arteries that feed your brain (so-called "vascular dementias") and cause strokes that can dramatically alter your cognitive abilities. Declining nerve function in your brain may also be linked to systemic inflammation and oxidative damage (caused by free radicals) that antioxidants work to control. The bottom line is that excellent blood sugar control helps keep your mind intact for all of these reasons, but poorer diabetes control can cause you to develop memory problems, vascular dementias, and possibly Alzheimer's disease.

The good news is that in many cases you can prevent these mental changes. All you need to do is eat better, exercise more, control your diabetes, smoke less, and frequently exercise your mind with challenging endeavors. For example, foods like blueberries and sweet potatoes with a lot of antioxidant power have been studied to determine if you're less likely to develop either dementia or Alzheimer's disease when you eat more of them, and it appears that they can actually help prevent these conditions. In addition, being overweight increases the risk of developing dementia at some point in your life, so keeping your weight in a more normal range is also beneficial. Almost all forms of physical activity improve insulin sensitivity and simultaneously decrease your risk of vascular changes that result in mental declines.

In addition, if you're mentally active throughout your lifetime, you will be significantly less likely to suffer declines in your mental capacity in your later years. In general, people who are more educated, have more intellectually challenging jobs, and engage in more mentally stimulating activities, such as attending lectures and plays, reading, playing chess, and doing hobbies, are much less likely to develop Alzheimer's and other forms of dementia. Scientists suspect that a lifetime of thinking a lot may create a cognitive reserve, a reservoir of brain power that you can draw upon even if you have a stroke or have protein deposits in your brain, a hallmark of Alzheimer's.

You will likely benefit most from engaging in a variety of stimulating activities. New experiences may be far more important than repeating the same task over and over, so try combining mental stimulation with social interaction for the greatest benefits. Most of all, you should enjoy the activities that you choose to take part in because stress and other negative emotions appear to be harmful to your mental abilities (not to mention your blood sugar control), and relaxation techniques may benefit your mental functioning for that reason. Even if you have the feeling your mental processes are already on the decline, you can still reverse the trend. Elderly people who go through training to sharpen their wits, for example, score much better on thinking tests for years afterward, and even the minds of younger people who continually drill their memories appear to work more efficiently. Peter Gariti likes to keep himself mentally challenged by signing up for continuing-education courses at nearby College of William & Mary in Williamsburg, Virginia.

Other longest-living people with diabetes have already adopted many of these suggestions as well. For instance, to keep her mind active and busy overall, Jo Allen plays bridge every Tuesday with her friends in Amarillo, Texas, and Robert Mandell also plays a lot of bridge over lunch. Blondie Fram keeps her mind working well by involving herself in more solitary, but equally mentally challenging, pursuits. "I never go to bed without doing a crossword puzzle—or Sudoku," she says. "People ask me if doing it right before bed keeps me awake, but when I'm tired, I can still go to sleep afterwards. I also read a lot, knit, and croquet. I'm always busy doing something." Zach Barneis also notes the importance of keeping active mentally.

MENTAL EXERCISES FOR MAINTENANCE OF A HEALTHIER, MORE VITAL MIND

- Practice memorizing anything and recall it later.
- Observe an object and then later draw it from memory.
- Draw a map or plan of places you have visited after you return home.
- Play card or board games that require more mental reasoning, such as pinochle, bridge, chess, checkers, or Othello.

- Do daily crossword puzzles, anagrams, Sudoku, and other word or reasoning games.
- Play video games, particularly the fast-moving ones that require quick reactions.
- Listen to or read the news and later on try to write down a summary.
- Try to do something new or unusual every day that requires you to think.
- Practice doing math problems in your head.
- Learn a new language, either on your own or by taking a class.
- Read a lot of different types of things, including fiction, nonfiction, and poetry.

Of all the people we interviewed for this book, including Gladys Dull, Gerald Cleveland, Bob Cleveland, Al Lewis, and all of the others with diabetes for longer than 50 years, not one exhibited any of the telltale symptoms of early dementia or significant memory loss. A great example of their collective functioning is Gerald Cleveland, who recently participated in a research study that found him to be the mental equivalent of a 20-year-old, even after 91 years of being alive and three-quarters of a century with diabetes. If you catch up with him, you'll quickly notice that he's always busy doing something, be it consulting with others about how to eat better to control blood sugar levels or being in charge of committees in his retirement community. All of these long-term diabetes survivors leave no doubt that an active body and a busy life lead to the maintenance of a fully functioning mind.

50

Do Everything in Moderation

The final secret of many long-time survivors is to practice moderation in all things, diabetes included. Moderation is defined by the internal battle between immediate gratification and self-control (i.e., resisting impulse). Does this mean that if you fail to adequately control your blood sugars one day you should give up trying to improve your diet and your health? Of course not! Consider a day lacking appropriate self-control to be the equivalent of "falling off the wagon" with drug or alcohol abuse. As long as you acknowledge your behavior and choose to get right back up on the wagon after your "fall," your health is not likely to suffer permanently.

Dan Spinazzola has a theory about most people with diabetes: He likens a diabetic individual in denial to an addicted cocaine user. "When a diabetic person's blood sugar is high, he says, 'Screw it. I'll eat a doughnut.' When he's low, he decides he needs a doughnut to treat it. When his blood sugars are good, he decides he's doing great and deserves a doughnut." As a person living with type 2 diabetes himself who tries hard but occasionally falls off his own wagon, he recognizes such thought patterns. "They also lie about what they're eating—both to others and to themselves. You have to be in the proper state of mind about diabetes. You can't be in denial about having it and expect to do well with it."

In most cases, complete abstinence from all temptations is unlikely to be the best way to make lifetime changes. For example, to maintain lifelong healthy eating, you don't need to completely abstain from any specific food. You can eat almost anything you want, as many long-time survivors do, with one big caveat: You simply need to learn or retrain yourself to consume unhealthier foods in moderation. This concept was introduced to Bernadette McIntyre early in her young life with diabetes. She recalls, "My mom still allowed me to enjoy some of the foods around the holidays. I just had small pieces of pie instead of full ones." When Robert Mandell was diagnosed with type 2 diabetes over 40 years ago, his doctor gave him similar advice. "He told me that he wasn't going to tell me not to eat pie," Robert says, "but rather just to make it a little piece. I still watch what I eat, and I eat a little bit of everything." Chuck Eichten agrees. The biggest thing he watches about his diet is the quantity of food that he's eating, although he admits that it's also important to understand food and what it can do for you and to you. "One bite of potato chips won't kill you," he says, "but you have to limit quantities. Just don't take in too much."

You can be assured that eating a dozen chocolate chip cookies at one sitting is not moderate, nor probably is consuming half a dozen. Moderation is eating one, maybe two (depending on their size, of course), and then you should monitor your blood sugars to keep them in control afterward rather than going into denial (and not treating any rise in your blood glucose) or counterproductively grappling with guilt over your actions. A good rule of thumb is that if the item you are splurging on affects your blood glucose levels at lot, you should limit yourself to only one small serving per day (or week or month).

You can also be more moderate by just taking a single bite of something you want rather than a whole serving. It's usually the first bite or two that tastes the best anyway. Also, eat it slowly and really savor it. Actually, you should do that with all the food you eat. Eating slowly allows your stomach to communicate with your brain through stretch receptors, and slower eating invariably results in earlier feelings of fullness. Drinking water or another fluid before a meal also has the same effect. Better yet, just plan a light snack for two to three hours after your meal instead of stuffing yourself at a meal. Dan Spinazzola admits that doing so is sometimes easier said than done. "My biggest barrier is my diet. I try to eat in moderation, but I'm from an Italian family, and I had lots of years of practice eating lots of breads and carbs, never leaving the table hungry, and eating lots of sweets. I could give up my wife before chocolate cookies!" Now there's a man who really loves his cookies.

Judy Tripathi admits she is moderate in her eating, not so much because of her diabetes, but simply because she's more concerned about her body weight. For Zach Barneis, forgetfulness is a problem. "I sometimes forget to bolus after eating," he says. Since it's an ongoing problem, he finally decided to start giving boluses with his insulin pump right before eating rather than waiting until afterward. "This also has the effect of making me stick to what I planned to eat," he says, "which helps my control. Do whatever it takes to convince yourself to do everything in moderation!"

Unless you have already given insulin to cover it (or you know your body can release enough), you should never feel obliged to finish all the food on your plate. It's much better to listen to your body's feedback about what it needs. As a general practice, eating to the point of feeling uncomfortably full should be avoided, as it's almost impossible to balance blood sugars in the short term when you eat too much (such as when trying to get your money's worth at an all-you-can-eat buffet). For better glucose control, you should probably avoid going to buffets or family-style restaurants, which are anything but moderate. If you have to eat at one and you can't order a separate à la carte meal instead, then first have a plateful of salad and vegetables and wait at least ten minutes before returning for a second, smaller plateful of entrée "samples." Never go back for a third helping, be sure to eat slowly, drink plenty of water during the meal, and try to stop eating when you're only about 80 percent full. Thus, when it comes to living long and well with a chronic disease like diabetes, your ability to focus more on your future health is critical in helping you make the right decisions to control your blood glucose levels now.

GERTRUDE "BLONDIE" FRAM, AGE 93, LIVING WITH TYPE 2 DIABETES FOR MORE THAN 40 YEARS

Blondie Fram has been living well with type 2 diabetes for at least four decades, but likely many more before she was diagnosed. She attributes her successes with diabetes first and foremost to her solid family support. "I have had wonderful support from my children and their spouses," she admits. Her success also comes in large part from the great medical support she has received, most of it coming from her son-in-law, Dr. Aaron I. Vinik, a world-renowned diabetologist and neuropathy specialist at the Strelitz Diabetes Institutes in Norfolk, Virginia. "In particular, my son-in-law has looked after me carefully. I know I could phone him in the middle of the night with any problem, but I try not to take advantage." After many years of controlling her diabetes with diet and exercise alone, he was instrumental in getting her on to insulin, which she takes currently four times a day.

A native of South Africa, she has always lived with one of her children and his or her family since she was widowed in her late 50s, and when they all immigrated to the United States, they brought her along with them. She currently spends six months with one of her daughters and her family in Nashville, Tennessee, and the other half of the year with her other daughter in Norfolk. It has been important for her to have her children around her all of that time, and she has also been able to help raise her grandchildren. "I think I've been really lucky to be surrounded by younger people all these years."

She's also a very active person who has refused to let life slow her down too much. She was a musician, and she still tries to get out to concerts. For years in South Africa, she played golf and tennis (even though ignorant practitioners in her home country tried to tell her that exercise is not good for people with diabetes). Until her last fall resulted in a bad fracture, she was walking in a local mall two to three miles a day. Now, she still tries to walk as much as possible because she knows how important being active is to living well—with or without diabetes. Her active lifestyle extends to mental exercise as well. She has always been a reader and belongs to a book club to this day. She never goes to bed without doing a crossword puzzle, and she also likes the Sudoku number puzzles. "You have to try to keep your mind going," she says, and it's apparent that this strategy has worked remarkably well for her.

Finally, Blondie also attributes her success at living well with diabetes to her positive outlook. "I always have something to look forward to. Right now I'm looking forward to seeing what colleges my great-grandkids get into!" She doesn't let her health problems bother her (she has been treated twice for breast cancer), and she is extremely careful with what she eats (a balanced diet with no added sugar and small quantities of food). "I have just learned to live with what I have to live with," she remarks. The fact that she can't move around as fast as she used to bothers her the most, but at 93 years old, she is still moving pretty fast.

Conclusion

A Last Few Words about Making the Secrets Work for You

Diabetes education and blood sugar control are still largely inadequate for most people living in the United States and around the world, and with the rapidly expanding cases of diabetes, we don't have to tell you that ignorance of how to prevent and control diabetes in this case is a very bad thing. Our primary goal with this book is to educate anyone who reads it. We want you, the reader, to know exactly what you need to do to take charge of your diabetic condition yourself and to be your own best advocate for better health and a longer life. Even if you're reading this for someone else (e.g., your child, parent, or other loved one), we want you to walk away with the conviction that a diagnosis of diabetes is not a reason to lose hope. In fact, with all the tools available to control diabetes that are available nowadays, you should be glad that you have this disease and not one of the less controllable ones!

Between the two of us, we have lived with diabetes longer than Gerald Cleveland has by himself (but collectively not as long as his brother Bob or Gladys Dull)—which is a humbling thought. Instead of saying to ourselves that we'll be lucky to live that long, after talking to all of these individuals, we're instead convinced that if they could do it, so can we. Similarly, we hope you have already learned a lot from the inspirational individuals living with type 1 and type 2 diabetes profiled in this book. In particular, the secrets given by the two Cleveland brothers sum up everything that you really need to focus on in order to live long and well with diabetes—and they should know, having more than 157 years of diabetes between them.

First of all, both of them placed physical activity as number one on their list of their top secrets to longevity (as did many other old-timers, along with Dr. Sheri). Bob Cleveland states, "Exercise is a definite priority for people with diabetes," and he advises people to get plenty of exercise, as he has done his entire life. Likewise, Gerald's top secret is simply, "Be active." Gladys Dull has been less active for the past several years due to health problems, but up until that time, she was always a very active person as well.

The Clevelands' second suggestion related to monitoring of blood sugars, with their individual advice being to "be aware of what you're doing" (Gerald) and to "keep a constant check on your blood glucose situation" (Bob). Doing so requires frequent blood glucose checks, along with vigilance about your dietary intake of carbs, fat, salt, and more that can affect your blood sugar, cholesterol levels, and overall health.

The third secret they both advocated involved a person's emotional state and outlook on life. Bob advises everyone to "live a good, clean life," replete with plenty of outdoor activities, a healthy diet, and a stable lifelong relationship. Gerald's comments are that he's "had a terrific life," and he makes this comment in spite of having had to deal with diabetes for 75 years, longer than most people live. Even according to the longest-living person of all, Gladys Dull, looking for the silver lining in any situation and appreciating what you do have instead of lamenting what you don't appear to be key to maintaining a positive outlook on life.

Finally, they both credit their longevity equally to their mother's diligent care when they were younger, as does Gladys Dull, and to advances in diabetes management over the past three-quarters of a century. "I marvel at being able to find out what my blood sugar is in only five seconds. There certainly have been great advances in diabetes care over the past 80 years!" says younger brother Bob. As Gerald says, "Have faith that the best things in life are ahead of you."

As for the rest of the old-timers living with diabetes for 40 or more years, their secrets most frequently emphasized the following items as being what they consider to be most important to their longevity with diabetes:

- Maintaining a positive attitude about diabetes and life in general
- Setting goals, particularly ones that are focused on having good health habits
- Learning all you can about diabetes and how to control it and its potential complications
- Having a supportive spouse, family, or friends, and involving other people in your diabetes care
- Sharing your diabetes with others or counseling them on how to live well with it
- Regularly monitoring your blood glucose levels
- Finding a good doctor, preferably an endocrinologist
- Always taking your insulin or other medications to control your blood sugars
- Watching your diet (whatever it may be), and keeping it healthy
- Exercising and staying as physically active as possible

Although none of these secrets is actually earth-shattering, taken as a whole, they do strongly suggest that certain behaviors are more important to longevity than others. Moreover, they emphasize the point that what people have to do to live a healthy, normal-length (or maybe longer-than-normal) life with diabetes is possible for anyone. Yes, you too can live long and well with any type of diabetes, just like all of the people profiled in this book are doing—and have done—day after day, year after year, decade after decade. If your blood sugars have not been that well controlled up to this point, you still can start reaping some of the health benefits of improving your control now. You may even be able to slow the progression of or reverse some of your complications with a little more diligence given to effectively managing your blood sugars. Diabetes care is rapidly changing nowadays, and there are new monitoring tools and medications to better control glycemic peaks and valleys. Most of the people who gave their secrets for this book have gone through a significant portion of their lives with this disease without the benefit of having all of these tools, or even adequate education, so think how much better you should be able to manage by having all of them at your disposal.

Today is the first day of the rest of your diabetic life. It's never too late to start taking better care of yourself, no matter if you have advanced complications or are new to diabetes. You have the power (and now the knowledge) to take control of your blood sugars once and for all. Our wish for every one of you is a long and healthy life with or without diabetes. Until there is a cure for this disease, just suffice it to say that it's possible—more than possible, maybe even probable—that you can and will live well and have a very long life. Actually, Dr. Sheri and Dr. Steve plan on living long enough with diabetes to ultimately die from something else! May the same rosy and largely realistic outcome be in your future.

ACKNOWLEDGMENTS

Without the assistance of the many people with diabetes who took the time to share their experiences with us, this book would not be all that it is today. We gratefully thank them for having lived long and well with diabetes to serve as inspirations to others living with diabetes. The knowledge they have collectively amassed is sure to help other people in ways we have yet to imagine, and they should feel proud.

We also owe thanks to our literary agent, Linda Konner, who heard about the incredible Cleveland brothers even before we did and suggested that their story would be a good basis for this book. Her belief in us and support throughout the creation of this book have been invaluable.

We would also like to gratefully acknowledge all of the industrious individuals at Marlowe & Company who have assisted all through the process. Our thanks particularly go to Matthew Lore, Marlowe's publisher and a fellow person with diabetes, whose encouragement and insight were critically important in shaping this book into its 50 secrets format (despite our initial reluctance to do so). We would also like to thank the other hardworking individuals at Marlowe & Company who have made this book a creation to behold, such as Courtney Napoles and others of whom we are probably not even aware.

Finally, we greatly appreciate the time that Etta Vinik took out of her incredibly busy schedule to read through the book and make suggestions that greatly enhanced its readability for everyone. We're lucky to have your invaluable support.

Our thanks go out to you all.

SUGGESTED READING

Becker, Gretchen. *The First Year—Type 2 Diabetes: An Essential Guide for the Newly Diagnosed.* 2nd ed. New York: Marlowe & Company, 2006.

Barnes, Darryl. *Action Plan for Diabetes: Your Guide to Controlling Blood Sugar.* Champaign, IL: Human Kinetics, 2004.

Brand-Miller, Jennie, et al. *The New Glucose Revolution.* 3rd ed. New York: Marlowe & Company, 2007.

Colberg, Sheri. *The Diabetic Athlete: Prescriptions for Exercise and Sports.* Champaign, IL: Human Kinetics, 2001.

Edelman, Steven V. *Taking Control of Your Diabetes.* 3rd ed. Caddo, OK: Professional Communications, Inc., 2007.

Hayes, Charlotte. *The "I Hate to Exercise" Book for People with Diabetes.* Alexandria, VA: American Diabetes Association, 2000.

Jackson, Richard, and Amy Tenderich. *Know Your Numbers, Outlive Your Diabetes: 5 Essential Health Factors You Can Master to Enjoy a Long and Healthy Life.* New York: Marlowe & Company, 2007.

Morley, John E., and Sheri R. Colberg. *Aging Successfully.* New York: McGraw-Hill, 2007.

Nathan, David, and Linda Delahanty. *Beating Diabetes (A Harvard Medical School Book).* New York: McGraw-Hill, 2005.

Peters, Anne. *Conquering Diabetes: A Cutting-Edge, Comprehensive Program for Prevention and Treatment.* New York: Hudson Street Press, 2005.

Price, Joan. *The Anytime, Anywhere Exercise Book.* Avon, MA: Adams Media Corporation, 2003.

Ruderman, Neil, ed. *Handbook of Exercise in Diabetes.* Alexandria, VA: American Diabetes Association, 2002.

Scheiner, Gary. *The Ultimate Guide to Accurate Carb Counting: Featuring the Tools and Techniques Used by the Experts.* New York: Marlowe & Company, 2007.

Scheiner, Gary. *Think Like a Pancreas: A Practical Guide to Managing Diabetes with Insulin.* New York: Marlowe & Company, 2004.

Warshaw, Hope. *The American Diabetes Association Guide to Healthy Restaurant Eating.* 3rd ed. Alexandria, VA: American Diabetes Association, 2005.

Warshaw, Hope. *What to Eat When You're Eating Out.* Alexandria, VA: American Diabetes Association, 2006.

SUGGESTED REFERENCES

Introduction

Centers for Disease Control and Prevention. 2000. National Diabetes Fact Sheet: General information and national estimates on diabetes in the United States, 2000. Retrieved from www.cdc.gov/diabetes/pubs/estimates.htm.

Hu, G., P. Jousilahti, N. C. Barengo, et al. 2005. Physical activity, cardiovascular risk factors, and mortality among Finnish adults with diabetes. *Diabetes Care* 28:799–805.

Narayan, K., J. Boyle, T. Thompson, et al. 2003. Lifetime risk for diabetes mellitus in the United States. *JAMA* 290:1884–1890.

Whiteley, L., S. Padmanabhan, D. Hole, et al. 2005. Should diabetes be considered a coronary heart disease risk equivalent? *Diabetes Care* 28:1588–1593.

Secret 1

Peyrot, M., J. F. McMurry, Jr., and D. F. Kruger. 1999. A biopsychosocial model of glycemic control in diabetes: stress, coping and regimen adherence. *J Health Soc Behav* 40(2):141–158.

Turan, B., Z. Osar, J. Molzan Turan, et al. 2002. The role of coping with disease in adherence to treatment regimen and disease control in type 1 and insulin treated type 2 diabetes mellitus. *Diabetes Metab* 28(3):186-193.

Secret 2

Begley, S. 2007. How the brain rewires itself. *Time* 169(5; January 29):72–79.

Brummett, B. H. , M. J. Helms, W. G. Dahlstrom, and I. C. Siegler. 2006. Prediction of all-cause mortality by the Minnesota Multiphasic Personality Inventory Optimism-Pessimism Scale scores: study of a college sample during a 40-year follow-up period. *Mayo Clin Proc* 81(12):1541–1544.

Rubin, R. R., and M. Peyrot. 2002. Was Willis right? Thoughts on the interaction of depression and diabetes. *Diabetes Metab Res Rev* 18(3):173–175.

Zhang, X., S. L. Norris, and E. W. Gregg, et al. 2005. Depressive symptoms and mortality among persons with and without diabetes. *Am J Epidemiol* 161:652–660.

Secret 3

Richardson, A., N. Adner, and G. Nordstrom. 2001. Persons with insulin-dependent diabetes mellitus: acceptance and coping ability. *J Adv Nurs* 33(6):758–763.

Snoek, F. J. 2002. Breaking the barriers to optimal glycaemic control: what physicians need to know from patients' perspectives. *Int J Clin Pract Suppl* (129):80–84.

Secret 4

Clark, A., A. Seidler, and M. Miller. 2001. Inverse association between sense of humor and coronary heart disease. *Int J Cardiol* 80(1):87–88.

Hayashi, K., T. Hayashi, S. Iwanaga, et al. 2003. Laughter lowered the increase in postprandial blood glucose. *Diabetes Care* 26(5):1651–1652.

Nasir, U. M., S. Iwanaga, A. H. Nabi, et al. 2005. Laughter therapy modulates the parameters of renin-angiotensin system in patients with type 2 diabetes. *Int J Mol Med* 16(6):1077–1081.

Secret 5

Attari, A., M. Sartippour, M. Amini, and S. Haghighi. 2006. Effect of stress management training on glycemic control in patients with type 1 diabetes. *Diabetes Res Clin Pract* 73(1):23–28.

Ciechanowski, P. S., W. J. Katon, and J. E. Russo. 2000. Depression and diabetes: impact of depressive symptoms on adherence, function, and costs. *Arch Intern Med* 160(21):3278–3285.

Gorman, C. 2007. 6 lessons for handling stress. *Time* 169(5; January 29):80–85.

Hartemann-Heurtier, A., S. Sultan, C. Sachon, et al. 2001. How type 1 diabetic patients with good or poor glycemic control cope with diabetes-related stress. *Diabetes Metab* 27(5; Paret 1):553–559.

Lucini, D., G. Di Fede, G. Parati, and M. Pagani. 2005. Impact of chronic psychosocial stress on autonomic cardiovascular regulation in otherwise healthy subjects. *Hypertension* 46(5):1201–1206.

Surwit, R. S., M. A. van Tilburg, N. Zucker, et al. 2002. Stress management improves long-term glycemic control in type 2 diabetes. *Diabetes Care* 25(1):30–34.

Taylor-Piliae, R. E., W. L. Haskell, C. M. Waters, and E. S. Froelicher. 2006.

Change in perceived psychosocial status following a 12-week Tai Chi exercise programme. *J Adv Nurs* 54(3):313–329.

Secret 6

Estabrooks, P. A., C. C. Nelson, S. Xu, et al. 2005. The frequency and behavioral outcomes of goal choices in the self-management of diabetes. *Diabetes Educ* 31(3):391–400.

Ilies, R. and T. A. Judge. 2005. Goal regulation across time: the effects of feedback and affect. *J Appl Psychol* 90(3):453–467.

Skinner, T. C. 2004. Psychological barriers. *Eur J Endocrinol* 151 Suppl 2:T13–17.

Sprague, M. A., J. A. Shultz, and L. J. Branen. 2006. Understanding patient experiences with goal setting for diabetes self-management after diabetes education. *Fam Community Health* 29(4):245–255.

Secret 7

Forlani, G., C. Zannoni, G. Tarrini et al. 2006. An empowerment-based educational program improves psychological well-being and health-related quality of life in Type 1 diabetes. *J Endocrinol Invest* 29(5):405–412.

Kavanagh, D. J., S. Gooley, and P. H. Wilson. 1993. Prediction of adherence and control in diabetes. *J Behav Med* 16(5):509–522.

Pibernik-Okanovic, M., M. Prasek, et al. 2004. Effects of an empowerment-based psychosocial intervention on quality of life and metabolic control in type 2 diabetic patients. *Patient Educ Couns 52* (2):193–199.

Rose, M., H. Fliege, M. Hildebrandt, et al. 2002. The network of psychological variables in patients with diabetes and their importance for quality of life and metabolic control. *Diabetes Care* 25(1):35–42.

Secret 8

Franciosi, M., F. Pellegrini, G. De Berardis, et al. 2001. The impact of blood glucose self-monitoring on metabolic control and quality of life in type 2 diabetic patients: an urgent need for better educational strategies. *Diabetes Care* 24(11):1870–1877.

Rafique, G., and F. Shaikh. 2006. Identifying needs and barriers to diabetes education in patients with diabetes. *J Pak Med Assoc* 56(8):347–352.

Schalch A. J., D. Ybarra, D. Adler, et al. 2001. Evaluation of a psycho-educational nutritional program in diabetic patients. *Patient Educ Couns* 44(2):171–178.

Tankova, T., G. Dakovska, and D. Koev. 2004. Education and quality of life in diabetic patients. *Patient Educ Couns,* 53(3):285–290.

Secret 9

Cheung, R., V. Young Cureton, and D. L. Canham. 2006. Quality of life in adolescents with type 1 diabetes who participate in diabetes camp. *J Sch Nurs* 22(1):53–58.

Karaguzel, G., I. Bircan, S. Erisir, and R. Bundak. 2005. Metabolic control and educational status in children with type 1 diabetes: effects of a summer camp and intensive insulin treatment. *Acta Diabetol* 42(4):156–161.

Keeter, E. L., and M. S. Linehan. 1993. Affecting children's attitudes toward diabetes through camp. *Nurse Pract* 18(8):25–26.

Secret 10

American Association of Diabetes Educators. 2002. Intensive diabetes management: implications of the DCCT and UKPDS. *Diabetes Educ* 28(5):735–740.

Dobretsov, M., D. Romanovsky, and J. R. Stimers. 2007. Early diabetic neuropathy: triggers and mechanisms. *World J Gastroenterol* 13(2):175–191.

Goldberg, R. B. 2003. Cardiovascular disease in patients who have diabetes. *Cardiol Clin* 21(3):399–413.

Nordwall, M., L. Hyllienmark, and J. Ludvigsson. 2006. Early diabetic complications in a population of young patients with type 1 diabetes mellitus despite intensive treatment. *J Pediatr Endocrinol Metab* 19(1):45–54.

Nathan, D. M., P. A. Cleary, J. Y. Backlund, et al. 2005. Intensive diabetes treatment and cardiovascular disease in patients with type 1 diabetes. *N Engl J Med* 353(25):2643–2653.

Secret 11

Laing, S. P., M. E. Jones, A. J. Swerdlow, et al. 2005. Psychosocial and socioeconomic risk factors for premature death in young people with type 1 diabetes. *Diabetes Care* 28(7):1618–1623.

Tankova, T., G. Dakovska, and D. Koev. 2001. Education of diabetic patients: a one year experience. *Patient Educ Couns* 43(2):139–145.

Vileikyte, L., R. R. Rubin, and H. Leventhal. 2004. Psychological aspects of diabetic neuropathic foot complications: an overview. *Diabetes Metab Res Rev* 20 Suppl 1:S13–18.

Secret 12

Balducci, S., G. Iacobellis, L. Parisi, et al. 2006. Exercise training can modify the natural history of diabetic peripheral neuropathy. *J Diabetes Complications* 20(4):216–223.

Hilpert, K. F., S. G. West, P. M. Kris-Etherton, et al. 2007. Postprandial effect of n-3 polyunsaturated fatty acids on apolipoprotein B-containing lipoproteins and vascular reactivity in type 2 diabetes. *Am J Clin Nutr* 85(2):369–376.

Hirsch, I. B. 2005. Intensifying insulin therapy in patients with type 2 diabetes mellitus. *Am J Med* 118 Suppl 5A:21S-26S.

Manley, S. 2003. Haemoglobin A1c: a marker for complications of type 2 diabetes: the experience from the UK Prospective Diabetes Study (UKPDS). *Clin Chem Lab Med* 41(9):1182–1190.

Nathan, D. M., J. Lachin, P. Cleary, et al. 2003. Intensive diabetes therapy and carotid intima-media thickness in type 1 diabetes mellitus. *N Engl J Med* 348(23):2294–2303,

Nicolucci, A., D. Cavaliere, N. Scorpiglione, et al. 1996. A comprehensive assessment of the avoidability of long-term complications of diabetes. A case-control study. SID-AMD Italian Study Group for the Implementation of the St. Vincent Declaration. *Diabetes Care* 19(9):927–933.

Pop-Busui, R., A. Sima, M. Stevens. 2006. Diabetic neuropathy and oxidative stress. *Diabetes Metab Res Rev* 22(4):257–273.

USDA Database for the Flavonoid Content of Selected Foods–2003. Accessed at www.nal.usda.gov/fnic/foodcomp/Data/Flav/flav.html on April 1, 2007.

Writing Team for the Diabetes Control and Complications Trial/Epidemiology of Diabetes Interventions and Complications Research Group. 2003. Sustained effect of intensive treatment of type 1 diabetes mellitus on development and progression of diabetic nephropathy: the Epidemiology of Diabetes Interventions and Complications (EDIC) study. *JAMA* 290(16):2159–2167.

Ziegler, D., A. Ametov, A. Barinov, et al. 2006. Oral treatment with alpha-lipoic acid improves symptomatic diabetic polyneuropathy: the SYDNEY 2 trial. *Diabetes Care* 29(11):2365–2370.

Secret 13

Davidson, J. 2005. Strategies for improving glycemic control: effective use of glucose monitoring. *Am J Med* 118(Suppl 9A):27S–32S.

Martin, S., B. Schneider, L. Heinemann, et al. 2006. Self-monitoring of blood glucose in type 2 diabetes and long-term outcome: an epidemiological cohort study. *Diabetologia* 49(2):271–278.

McCarter, R. J., J. M. Hempe, S. A. Chalew. 2006. Mean blood glucose and biological variation have greater influence on HbA1c levels than glucose instability: an analysis of data from the Diabetes Control and Complications Trial. *Diabetes Care* 29(2):352–355.

Murata, G. H., J. H. Shah, R. M. Hoffman, et al. 2003. Intensified blood glucose monitoring improves glycemic control in stable, insulin-treated veterans with type 2 diabetes: the Diabetes Outcomes in Veterans Study (DOVES). *Diabetes Care* 26(6):1759–1763.

Puder, J. J., J. Endrass, N. Moriconi, and U. Keller. 2006. How patients with insulin-treated type 1 and type 2 diabetes view their own and their physician's treatment goals. *Swiss Med Wkly* 136(35–36):574–580.

Secret 14

Ceriello, A. 2003. The possible role of postprandial hyperglycaemia in the pathogenesis of diabetic complications. *Diabetologia* 46 Suppl 1:M9–16.

Hirsch, I. B., and M. Brownlee. 2005. Should minimal blood glucose variability become the gold standard of glycemic control? *J Diabetes Complications* 19(3):178–181.

Schutt, M., W. Kern, U. Krause, et al. 2006. Is the frequency of self-monitoring of blood glucose related to long-term metabolic control? Multicenter analysis including 24,500 patients from 191 centers in Germany and Austria. *Exp Clin Endocrinol Diabetes* 114(7):384–388.

Ziegher, O., M. Kolopp, J. Louis J, et al. 1993. Self-monitoring of blood glucose and insulin dose alteration in type 1 diabetes mellitus. *Diabetes Res Clin Pract* 21(1):51–59.

Secret 15

Bischof, M. G., E. Bernroider, C. Ludwig, et al. 2001. Effect of near physiologic insulin therapy on hypoglycemia counterregulation in type-1 diabetes. *Horm Res* 56(5–6):151–158,

Cryer, P. E. 2006. Hypoglycemia in diabetes: pathophysiological mechanisms and diurnal variation. *Prog Brain Res* 153:361–365.

Cryer, P. E. 2002. Hypoglycaemia: the limiting factor in the glycaemic management of Type I and Type II diabetes. *Diabetologia* 45(7):937–948.

Davis, S., and M. D. Alonso. 2004. Hypoglycemia as a barrier to glycemic control. *J Diabetes Complications* 18(1):60–68.

DeVries, J. H., I. M. Wentholt, N. Masurel, et al. 2004. Nocturnal hypoglycaemia in type 1 diabetes: consequences and assessment. *Diabetes Metab Res Rev* 20 Suppl 2:S43–46.

Edelman, S. V., and C. M. Morello. 2004. Hypoglycemia unawareness and type 1 diabetes. *South Med J* 97(11):1143–1144.

Gomis, R., and E. Esmatjes. 2004. Asymptomatic hypoglycaemia: identification and impact. *Diabetes Metab Res Rev* 20 Suppl 2:S47–49.

Graveling, A. J., R. E. Warren, and B. M. Frier. 2004. Hypoglycaemia and driving in people with insulin-treated diabetes: adherence to recommendations for avoidance. *Diabet Med* 21(9):1014–1019.

Henderson J. N., K. V. Allen, I. J. Deary, and B. M. Frier. 2003. Hypogly-caemia in insulin-treated Type 2 diabetes: frequency, symptoms and impaired awareness. *Diabet Med* 20(12):1016–1021.

Nordfeldt, S., and J. Ludvigsson. 2005. Fear and other disturbances of severe hypoglycaemia in children and adolescents with type 1 diabetes mellitus. *J Pediatr Endocrinol Metab* 18(1):83–91.

Sandoval, D. A., D. L. Guy, M. A. Richardson, et al. 2006. Acute, same-day effects of antecedent exercise on counterregulatory responses to subsequent hypoglycemia in type 1 diabetes mellitus. *Am J Physiol Endocrinol Metab* 290(6):E1331–1338.

Secret 16

Brand-Miller, J., S. Hayne, P. Petocz, and S. Colagiuri. 2003. Low-glycemic index diets in the management of diabetes: A meta-analysis of randomized control trials. *Diabetes Care* 26:2261–2267.

Foster-Powell, K., S. Holt, and J. Brand-Miller. 2002. International table of glycemic index and glycemic load values: 2002. *Am J Clin Nutr* 76:5–56.

Hernandez, J. M., T. Moccia, J. D. Fluckey, et al. 2000. Fluid snacks to help persons with type 1 diabetes avoid late onset postexercise hypoglycemia. *Med Sci Sports Exerc* 32 (5):904–910.

Secret 17

Brackenridge, A., H. Wallbank, R. A. Lawrenson, and D. Russell-Jones. 2006. Emergency management of diabetes and hypoglycaemia. *Emerg Med J* 23(3):183–185.

Hartley, M., M. J. Thomsett, and A. M. Cotterill. 2006. Mini-dose glucagon rescue for mild hypoglycaemia in children with type 1 diabetes: the Bris-bane experience. *J Paediatr Child Health* 42(3):108–111.

Suh S. W., K. Aoyama, Y. Matsumori, et al. 2005. Pyruvate administered after severe hypoglycemia reduces neuronal death and cognitive impairment. *Diabetes* 54(5):1452–1458.

Secret 18

Ciechanowski, P. S., W. J. Katon, J. E. Russo, and E. A. Walker. 2001. The patient-provider relationship: attachment theory and adherence to treat-ment in diabetes. *Am J Psychiatry* 158(1):29–35.

Nguyen, T. T., N. A. Daniels, G. L. Gildengorin, and E. J. Perez-Stable. 2007. Ethnicity, language, specialty care, and quality of diabetes care. *Ethn Dis* 17(1):65–71.

Yun, K. E., M. J. Park, and H. S. Park, 2007. Lack of management of cardio-vascular risk factors in type 2 diabetic patients. *Int J Clin Pract* 61(1):39–44.

Secret 19

Arora, S. K., and S. I. McFarlane. 2005. The case for low carbohydrate diets in diabetes management. *Nutr Metab* (Lond), 2:16.

Brand-Miller, J., S. Hayne, P. Petocz, and S. Colagiuri. 2003. Low-glycemic index diets in the management of diabetes: A meta-analysis of randomized control trials. *Diabetes Care* 26:2261–2267.

Foster-Powell, K., S. Holt, and J. Brand-Miller. 2002. International table of glycemic index and glycemic load values: 2002. *Am J Clin Nutr* 76:5–56.

Grassi, D., C. Lippi, S. Necozione, et al. 2005. Short-term administration of dark chocolate is followed by a significant increase in insulin sensitivity and a decrease in blood pressure in healthy persons. *Am J Clin Nutr* 81:611–614.

Liu, R. 2003. Health benefits of fruit and vegetables are from additive and synergistic combinations of phytochemicals. *Am J Clin Nutr* 78:517S–520S.

Lovejoy, J. 2002. The influence of dietary fat on insulin resistance. *Curr Diabetes Reports* 2:435–440.

Qi, L., R. M. van Dam, S. Liu, et al. 2006. Whole-grain, bran, and cereal fiber intakes and markers of systemic inflammation in diabetic women. *Diabetes Care* 29(2):207-211.

Slama, G., F. Elgrably, M. Kabir, and S. Rizkalla. 2006. Low glycemic index foods should play a role in improving overall glycemic control in type-1 and type-2 diabetic patients and, more specifically, in correcting excessive postprandial hyperglycemia. *Nestle Nutr Workshop Ser Clin Perform Programme* 11:73–81.

Wolever, T. M., S. Hamad, J. L. Chiasson, et al. 1999. Day-to-day consistency in amount and source of carbohydrate associated with improved blood glucose control in type 1 diabetes. *J Am Coll Nutr* 18(3):242–247.

Secret 20

Chiesa, G., M. A. Piscopo, A. Rigamonti, et al. 2005. Insulin therapy and carbohydrate counting. *Acta Biomed* 76 Suppl 3:44–48.

Gillespie, S. J., K. D. Kulkarni, and A. E. Daly. 1998. Using carbohydrate counting in diabetes clinical practice. *J Am Diet Assoc* 98(8):897–905.

Wolever, T. M., S. Hamad, J. L. Chiasson, et al. 1999. Day-to-day consistency in amount and source of carbohydrate associated with improved blood glucose control in type 1 diabetes. *J Am Coll Nutr* 18(3):242-247.

Secret 21

Brand-Miller, J., S. Hayne, P. Petocz, and S. Colagiuri. 2003. Low-glycemic index diets in the management of diabetes: A meta-analysis of randomized control trials. *Diabetes Care* 26:2261–2267.

Burani, J., and P. J. Longo. 2006. Low-glycemic index carbohydrates: an effective behavioral change for glycemic control and weight management in patients with type 1 and 2 diabetes. *Diabetes Educ* 32(1):78–88.

Galgani, J., C. Aguirre, and E. Diaz. 2006. Acute effect of meal glycemic index and glycemic load on blood glucose and insulin responses in humans. *Nutr J* 5:22.

Kelley, D. E. Sugars and starch in the nutritional management of diabetes mellitus. 2003. *Am J Clin Nutr* 78(4):858S–864S.

Secret 22

Bove, A., J. Hebreo, J. Wylie-Rosett, and C. R. Isasi. 2006. Burger King and Subway: key nutrients, glycemic index, and glycemic load of nutritionally promoted items. *Diabetes Educ* 32(5):675–690.

Pereira, M. A., A. I. Kartashov, C. B. Ebbeling, et al. Fast-food habits, weight gain, and insulin resistance (the CARDIA study): 15-year prospective analysis. *Lancet* 365(9453):36–42, 2005.

Vlachokosta, F. V., C. M. Piper, R. Gleason, et al. 1988. Dietary carbohydrate, a Big Mac, and insulin requirements in type I diabetes. *Diabetes Care* 11(4):330–336.

Warshaw, H. S. Fast food and restaurant fare. 2002. Nutrition tips. On estimating portion sizes. *Diabetes Forecast* 55(5):55–57.

Warshaw, Hope. 2005. The American Diabetes Association Guide to Healthy Restaurant Eating. 3rd edition. Alexandria, VA: American Diabetes Association.

Warshaw, Hope. 2006. What to Eat When You're Eating Out. Alexandria, VA: American Diabetes Association.

Webb, R. 2006. On the road again. Food fit for traveling. *Diabetes Forecast* 59(2):20, 22, 24.

Secret 23

Levy-Marchal, C., K. Perlman, B. Zinman, et al. 1986. Preprogrammed intravenous insulin infusion in diabetic humans: metabolic consequences of altering meal size. *Diabetes Care* 9(3):283–290.

Powell, J. T., P. J. Franks, and N. R. Poulter. 1999. Does nibbling or grazing protect the peripheral arteries from atherosclerosis? *J Cardiovasc Risk* 6(1):19–22.

Vlachokosta, F. V., C. M. Piper, R. Gleason, et al. 1988. Dietary carbohydrate, a Big Mac, and insulin requirements in type I diabetes. *Diabetes Care* 11(4):330–336.

Secret 24

Al-Shammari, K. F., J. M. Al-Ansari, N. M. Moussa, et al. 2006. Association of periodontal disease severity with diabetes duration and diabetic complications in patients with type 1 diabetes mellitus. *J Int Acad Periodontol.* 8(4):109–114.

Briggs, J. E, P. P. McKeown, V. L. Crawford, et al. 2006. Angiographically confirmed coronary heart disease and periodontal disease in middle-aged males. *J Periodontol* 77(1):95–102.

Hyman, J. J., D. M. Winn, and B. C. Reid. 2002. The role of cigarette smoking in the association between periodontal disease and coronary heart disease. *J Periodontol* 73(9):988–994.

Mealey, B. L., T. W. Oates; American Academy of Periodontology. 2006. Diabetes mellitus and periodontal diseases. *J Periodontol* 77(8):1289–1303.

Secret 25

Berggren, J. R., M. W. Hulver, and J. A. Houmard. 2005. Fat as an endocrine organ: influence of exercise. *J Appl Physiol* 99(2):757–764.

Borghouts, L., and H. Keizer. 2000. Exercise and insulin sensitivity: A review. *Int J Sports Med* 21:1–12.

Bruce, C., and J. Hawley. 2004. Improvements in insulin resistance with aerobic exercise training: A lipocentric approach. *Med Sci Sports Exerc* 36:1196–1201.

Ertl, A. C., S. N. Davis. 2004. Evidence for a vicious cycle of exercise and hypoglycemia in type 1 diabetes mellitus. *Diabetes Metab Res Rev* 20(2):124–130.

Koivisto, V. A., T. Sane, F. Fyhrquist, and R. Pelkonen. 1992. Fuel and fluid homeostasis during long-term exercise in healthy subjects and type I diabetic patients. *Diabetes Care* 15(11):1736–1741.

Secret 26

De Feo, P., C. Di Loreto, A. Ranchelli, et al. 2006. Exercise and diabetes. *Acta Biomed* 77 Suppl 1:14–17.

Di Loreto, C., C. Fanelli, P. Lucidi, et al. 2005. Make your diabetic patients walk: Long-term impact of different amounts of physical activity on type 2 diabetes. *Diabetes Care* 28:1295–1302.

Engel, L., and H. Lindner. 2006. Impact of using a pedometer on time spent walking in older adults with type 2 diabetes. *Diabetes Educ* 32(1):98–107.

Houmard, J. A., C. J. Tanner, C. A. Slentz, et al. 2004. Effect of the volume and intensity of exercise training on insulin sensitivity. *J Appl Physiol* 96:101–106.

Hultquist, C. N., C. Albright, D. L. Thompson. 2005. Comparison of walking recommendations in previously inactive women. *Med Sci Sports Exerc* 37:676–683.

Kubukeli, Z. N, T. D. Noakes, S. C. Dennis. 2002. Training techniques to improve endurance exercise performances. *Sports Med* 32:489–509.

Penedo, F. J., and J. R. Dahn. 2005. Exercise and well-being: a review of mental and physical health benefits associated with physical activity. *Curr Opin Psychiatry* 18(2):189–193.

Secret 27

Bergman, B. C., G. E. Butterfield, E. E. Wolfel, et al. 1999. Muscle net glucose uptake and glucose kinetics after endurance training in men. *Am J Physiol* 277(1 Pt 1):E81-92.

Bruce, C., and J. Hawley. 2004. Improvements in insulin resistance with aerobic exercise training: A lipocentric approach. *Med Sci Sports Exerc* 36:1196–1201.

Bussau, V. A., L. D. Ferreira, T. W. Jones, and P. A. Fournier. 2006. The 10-s maximal sprint: a novel approach to counter an exercise-mediated fall in glycemia in individuals with type 1 diabetes. *Diabetes Care* 29(3):601–606.

Johnson, S. T., L. J. McCargar, G. J. Bell, C. Tudor-Locke, V. J. Harber, and R. C. Bell. 2006. Walking faster: distilling a complex prescription for type 2 diabetes management through pedometry. *Diabetes Care* 29(7):1654–1655.

Secret 28

Brubaker, P. L. 2005. Adventure travel and type 1 diabetes: the complicating effects of high altitude. *Diabetes Care* 28(10):2563–2572.

Fahey, P. J., E. T. Stallkamp, and S. Kwatra. 1996. The athlete with type I diabetes: managing insulin, diet and exercise. *Am Fam Physician* 53(5):1611–1624.

Koivisto, V. A., T. Sane, F. Fyhrquist, and R. Pelkonen. 1992. Fuel and fluid homeostasis during long-term exercise in healthy subjects and type I diabetic patients. *Diabetes Care* 15(11):1736–1741.

Lisle, D. K., and T. H. Trojian. 2006. Managing the athlete with type 1 diabetes. *Curr Sports Med Rep* 5(2):93–98.

Secret 29

Bonen, A., G. L. Dohm, L. J. van Loon. 2006. Lipid metabolism, exercise and insulin action. *Essays Biochem* 42:47–59.

Borghouts, L, and H. Keizer. 2000. Exercise and insulin sensitivity: A review. *Int J Sports Med* 21:1–12.

Bruce, C., J. Hawley. 2004. Improvements in insulin resistance with aerobic exercise training: A lipocentric approach. *Med Sci Sports Exerc* 36:1196–1201,

Henriksen, E. J. 2006. Exercise training and the antioxidant alpha-lipoic acid in the treatment of insulin resistance and type 2 diabetes. *Free Radic Biol Med* 40(1):3–12.

Pedersen, B. K., and B. Saltin. 2006. Evidence for prescribing exercise as therapy in chronic disease. *Scand J Med Sci Sports* 16 Suppl 1:3–63.

Secret 30

Albu, J., and N. Raja-Khan. 2003. The management of the obese diabetic patient. *Prim Care* 30(2):465–491.

Astrup, A. 2006. How to maintain a healthy body weight. *Int J Vitam Nutr Res* 76(4):208–215.

Burani, J., and P. J. Longo. 2006. Low-glycemic index carbohydrates: an effective behavioral change for glycemic control and weight management in patients with type 1 and 2 diabetes. *Diabetes Educ* 32(1):78–88.

Giannopoulou, I., L. L. Ploutz-Synder, R. Carhart, et al. 2005. Exercise is required for visceral fat loss in postmenopausal women with type 2 diabetes. *J Clin Endo Metab* 90:1511–1518.

Hamman, R. F., R. R. Wing, S. L. Edelstein, et al. 2006. Effect of weight loss with lifestyle intervention on risk of diabetes. *Diabetes Care* 29(9):2102–2107.

Muis, M. J., M. L. Bots, H. J. Bilo, et al. 2006. Determinants of daily insulin use in Type 1 diabetes. *J Diabetes Complications,* 20(6):356-360.

Sibley, S. D., J. P. Palmer, I. B. Hirsch, and J. D. Brunzell. 2003. Visceral obesity, hepatic lipase activity, and dyslipidemia in type 1 diabetes. *J Clin Endocrinol Metab* 88(7):3379–3384.

Secret 31

Davis, S. N., and S. M. Renda. 2006. Psychological insulin resistance: overcoming barriers to starting insulin therapy. *Diabetes Educ* 32 Suppl 4:146S–152S.

Garg, S. K., S. L. Ellis, and H. Ulrich. 2005. Insulin glulisine: a new rapid-acting insulin analogue for the treatment of diabetes. *Expert Opin Pharmacother* 6(4):643–651.

Peterson, G. E. 2006. Intermediate and long-acting insulins: a review of NPH insulin, insulin glargine and insulin detemir. *Curr Med Res Opin* 22(12):2613–2619.

Polonsky, W. H., B. J. Anderson, P. A. Lohrer, et al. 1994. Insulin omission in women with IDDM. *Diabetes Care* 17(10):1178–1185.

Raskin, P., E. Allen, P. Hollander, et al. 2005. Initiating insulin therapy in type

2 Diabetes: a comparison of biphasic and basal insulin analogs. *Diabetes Care* 28(2):260–265.

Rave, K., S. Bott, L. Heinemann, et al. 2005. Time-action profile of inhaled insulin in comparison with subcutaneously injected insulin lispro and regular human insulin. *Diabetes Care* 28:1077–1082.

Secret 32

de Galan, B. E. 2004. Insulin pump therapy, should we consider it more often? *Neth J Med* 62(10):341–343.

Everett, J. 2004. The role of insulin pumps in the management of diabetes. *Nurs Times* 100(16):48–49.

Herman, W. H., L. L. Ilag, S. L. Johnson, et al. 2005. A clinical trial of continuous subcutaneous insulin infusion versus multiple daily injections in older adults with type 2 diabetes. *Diabetes Care* 28(7):1568–1573.

Linkeschova, R., M. Raoul, U. Bott, et al. 2002. Less severe hypoglycaemia, better metabolic control, and improved quality of life in Type 1 diabetes mellitus with continuous subcutaneous insulin infusion (CSII) therapy; an observational study of 100 consecutive patients followed for a mean of 2 years. *Diabet Med* 19(9):746–751.

Scheiner G. Go ahead, pick your pump. 2006. Which pump is right for you? *Diabetes Self Manag* 23(6):12, 14 16, 19–20.

Secret 33

Bond, A. 2006. Exenatide (Byetta) as a novel treatment option for type 2 diabetes mellitus. Proc (Bayl Univ Med Cent), 19(3):281–284.

Green, B. D., R. R. Flatt, C. J. Bailey. 2006. Dipeptidyl peptidase IV (DPP IV) inhibitors: A newly emerging drug class for the treatment of type 2 diabetes. *Diab Vasc Dis Res* 3(3):159–165.

Joy, S. V., P. T. Rodgers, and A. C. Scates. 2005. Incretin mimetics as emerging treatment for type 2 diabetes. *Ann Pharmacotherapy* 39:110–118.

Moon, R. J., L. A. Bascombe, and R. I. Holt. 2007. The addition of metformin in type 1 diabetes improves insulin sensitivity, diabetic control, body composition and patient well-being. *Diabetes Obes Metab* 9(1):143–145.

Secret 34

Arabadjief, D., and J. H. Nichols. Assessing glucose meter accuracy. 2006. *Curr Med Res Opin* 22(11):2167–2174.

Karter, A. J. 2006. Role of self-monitoring of blood glucose in glycemic control. *Endocr Pract* 12 Suppl 1:110–117.

Mensing, C. 2004. Helping patients choose the right blood glucose meter. *Nurse Pract* 29(5):43–45.

Roberts, S. S. 2005. Choosing a meter. Pick one that's right for you. *Diabetes Forecast* 58(10):35–36.

Sarol, J. N., Jr., N. A. Nicodemus, Jr., K. M. Tan, and M. B. Grava. 2005. Self-monitoring of blood glucose as part of a multi-component therapy among non-insulin requiring type 2 diabetes patients: a meta-analysis (1966–2004). *Curr Med Res Opin* 21(2):173–184.

Schutt, M., W. Kern, U. Krause, et al. 2006. Is the frequency of self-monitoring of blood glucose related to long-term metabolic control? Multicenter analysis including 24,500 patients from 191 centers in Germany and Austria. *Exp Clin Endocrinol Diabetes* 114(7):384–388.

Secret 35

Deiss, D., R. Hartmann, J. Hoeffe, and O. Kordonouri. 2004. Assessment of glycemic control by continuous glucose-monitoring system in 50 children with type 1 diabetes starting on insulin pump therapy. *Pediatr Diabetes* 5(3):117–121.

Garg S, and L. Jovanovic. 2006. Relationship of fasting and hourly blood glucose levels to HbA1c values: safety, accuracy, and improvements in glucose profiles obtained using a 7-day continuous glucose sensor. *Diabetes Care* 29(12):2644–2649.

Kruger, D., and A. O. Marcus. 2000. Psychological motivation and patient education: a role for continuous glucose monitoring. *Diabetes Technol Ther* 2 Suppl 1:S93-97.

McCall, A. L., D. J. Cox, J. Crean, et al. 2006. A novel analytical method for assessing glucose variability: using CGMS in type 1 diabetes mellitus. *Diabetes Technol Ther* 8(6):644–653.

Secret 36

Juvenile Diabetes Research Foundation International. Clinical Trials. Accessed at www.jdrf.org/index.cfm?page_id=101984.

NIH Resource Information on Clinical Trials. Accessed at www.clinicaltrials.gov/ct/info/resources.

Rosen, E. D. Participation in clinical trials. Accessed at www.diabetes.org/diabetes-research/clinical-trials/trials-home.jsp.

Steffes, M., P. Cleary, D. Goldstein, et al. 2005. Hemoglobin A1c measurements over nearly two decades: sustaining comparable values throughout the Diabetes Control and Complications Trial and the Epidemiology of Diabetes Interventions and Complications study. *Clin Chem* 51(4):753–758.

Veritas Medicine: About Clinical Trials. Accessed February 2007 at www.veri-tasmedicine.com/about_trials.cfm?frm=fm.

Secret 37

Graue, M., T. Wentzel-Larsen, B. R. Hanestad, and O. Sovik. 2005. Health-related quality of life and metabolic control in adolescents with diabetes: the role of parental care, control, and involvement. *J Pediatr Nurs* 20(5):373–382.

van Dam, H. A., F. G. van der Horst, L. Knoops, et al. 2005. Social support in diabetes: a systematic review of controlled intervention studies. *Patient Educ Couns* 59(1):1–12.

Secret 38

Gilden, J. L., M. S. Hendryx, S. Clar, et al. 1992. Diabetes support groups improve health care of older diabetic patients. *J Am Geriatr Soc* 40(2):147–150.

McPherson, S. L., D. Joseph, and E. Sullivan. 2004. The benefits of peer support with diabetes. *Nurs Forum* 39(4):5–12.

Pector, E. A. 2004. Online diabetes support groups. *Diabetes Self Manag* 21(2):95, 97–99.

van Dam, H. A., F. G. van der Horst, L. Knoops, et al. 2005. Social support in diabetes: a systematic review of controlled intervention studies. *Patient Educ Couns* 59(1):1–12.

Secret 39

Graue, M., T. Wentzel-Larsen, B. R. Hanestad, and O. Sovik. 2005. Health-related quality of life and metabolic control in adolescents with diabetes: the role of parental care, control, and involvement. *J Pediatr Nurs* 20(5):373–382.

Konen, J. C., J. H. Summerson, and M. B. Dignan. 1993. Family function, stress, and locus of control. Relationships to glycemia in adults with diabetes mellitus. *Arch Fam Med* 2(4):393–402.

Trief, P. M., R. Ploutz-Snyder, K. D. Britton, and R. S. Weinstock. 2004. The relationship between marital quality and adherence to the diabetes care regimen. *Ann Behav Med* 27(3):148–154.

Trief, P. M., M. J. Wade, K. D. Britton, and R. S. Weinstock. 2002. A prospective analysis of marital relationship factors and quality of life in diabetes. *Diabetes Care* 25(7):1154–1158.

Secret 40

Baker J., R. Scragg, P. Metcalf, and E. Dryson. 1993. Diabetes mellitus and employment: is there discrimination in the workplace? *Diabet Med* 10(4):362–365.

Griffiths, R. D., and R. G. Moses. 1993. Diabetes in the workplace. Employment experiences of young people with diabetes mellitus. *Med J Aust* 158(3):169–171.

McMahon, B. T., S. L. West, M. Mansouri, and L. Belongia. 2005. Workplace discrimination and diabetes: the EEOC Americans with Disabilities Act research project. *Work* 25(1):9–18.

Secret 41

Powers, M. A., and M. L. Wheeler. 1993. Model for dietetics practice and research: the challenge is here, but the journey was not easy. *J Am Diet Assoc* 93(7):755–757.

Silverstein, J. H., and R. Bandyopadhyay. 1995. Camping with a friend. Helping adolescents cope with diabetes. *J Fla Med Assoc* 82(12):817–820.

Secret 42

Jensen, D. M., P. Damm, L. Moelsted-Pedersen, et al. 2004. Outcomes in type 1 diabetic pregnancies: a nationwide, population-based study. *Diabetes Care* 27(12):2819–2823.

McElvy, S. S., M. Miodovnik, B. Rosenn, et al. 2000. A focused preconceptional and early pregnancy program in women with type 1 diabetes reduces perinatal mortality and malformation rates to general population levels. *J Matern Fetal Med* 9(1):14–20.

Verier-Mine, O., N. Chaturvedi, D. Webb, and J. H. Fuller. 2005. Is pregnancy a risk factor for microvascular complications? *The EURODIAB Prospective Complications Study. Diabet Med* 22(11):1503–1509.

Secret 43

American Diabetes Association. When you Travel. Accessed at www.diabetes.org/pre-diabetes/travel/when-you-travel.jsp.

American Diabetes Association. Traveling with diabetes supplies. Accessed at www.diabetes.org/advocacy-and-legalresources/discrimination/public_accommodation/travel.jsp

Dairman, T. 2006. Diabetes resources. Travel tips. *Diabetes Self Manag* 23(4):64–65.

Kruger, Davida F. 2001. The Diabetes Travel Guide: How to Travel with Diabetes Anywhere in the World. Alexandria, VA: American Diabetes Association.

Lumber, T., and P. A. Strainic. 2005. Have insulin, will travel. Planning ahead will make traveling with insulin smooth sailing. *Diabetes Forecast* 58(8):50–54.

Secret 44

Brooks, F., and J. Magnusson. 2006. Taking part counts: adolescents' experiences of the transition from inactivity to active participation in school-based physical education. *Health Educ Res* 21(6):872–883.

Verghese, J. 2006. Cognitive and mobility profile of older social dancers. *J Am Geriatr Soc* 54(8):1241–1244.

Secret 45

Raina, P., D. Waltner-Toews, B. Bonnett, C. Woodward, and T. Abernathy. 1999. Influence of companion animals on the physical and psychological health of older people: an analysis of a one-year longitudinal study. *J Am Geriatr Soc* 47(3):323–329.

Voelker, R. 2006. Studies suggest dog walking a good strategy for fostering fitness. *JAMA* 296(6):643.

Secret 46

Henderson, J. N., K. V. Allen, I. J. Deary, and B. M. Frier. 2003. Hypoglycaemia in insulin-treated Type 2 diabetes: frequency, symptoms and impaired awareness. *Diabet Med* 20(12):1016–1021.

Polonsky, W. H., C. L. Davis, A. M. Jacobson, and B. J. Anderson. 1992. Hyperglycaemia, hypoglycaemia, and blood glucose control in diabetes: symptom perceptions and treatment strategies. *Diabet Med* 9(2):120–125.

Warren, R. E., I. J. Deary, B. M. Frier. 2003. The symptoms of hyperglycaemia in people with insulin-treated diabetes: classification using principal components analysis. *Diabetes Metab Res Rev* 19(5):408–414.

Secret 47

Fanelli, C., S. Pampanelli, C. Lalli, et al. 1997. Long-term intensive therapy of IDDM patients with clinically overt autonomic neuropathy: effects on hypoglycemia awareness and counterregulation. *Diabetes* 46(7):1172–1181.

Gignac, M. A., A. M. Davis, G. Hawker, et al. 2006. "What do you expect? You're just getting older": A comparison of perceived osteoarthritis-related and aging-related health experiences in middle- and older-age adults. *Arthritis Rheum* 55(6):905–912.

Heise, T., T. Koschinsky, L. Heinemann, et al. 2003. Hypoglycemia warning signal and glucose sensors: requirements and concepts. *Diabetes Technol Ther,* 5(4):563–571.

Widom, B, M. P. Diamond, and D. C. Simonson. 1992. Alterations in glucose metabolism during menstrual cycle in women with IDDM. *Diabetes Care* 15(2):213–220.

Secret 48

De Cosmo, S., O. Lamacchia, A. Rauseo, et al. 2006. Cigarette smoking is associated with low glomerular filtration rate in male patients with type 2 diabetes. *Diabetes Care* 29(11):2467–2470.

Eliasson, B. 2003. Cigarette smoking and diabetes. *Prog Cardiovasc Dis* 45(5):405–413.

Wynd, C. A. 2006. Smoking patterns, beliefs, and the practice of healthy behaviors in abstinent, relapsed, and recalcitrant smokers. *Appl Nurs Res* 19(4):197–203.

Secret 49

Banks, W. A., and J. E. Morley. 2003. Memories are made of this: Recent advances in understanding cognitive impairments and dementia. *J Gerontol* 58(4):314–321.

Cukierman, T., H. C. Gerstein, and J. D. Williamson. 2005. Cognitive decline and dementia in diabetes-systematic overview of prospective observational studies. *Diabetologia* 48(12):2460–2469.

Fox, K. R. 1999. The influence of physical activity on mental well-being. *Public Health Nutr* 2(3A):411–418.

Secret 50

Jebb, S. A. 2005. Dietary strategies for the prevention of obesity. *Proc Nutr Soc* 64(2):217–227.

Wadden, T. A., M. L. Butryn, and K. J. Byrne. 2004. Efficacy of lifestyle modification for long-term weight control. *Obes Res* 12 Suppl:151S–162S.

Young, L. R., and M. Nestle. 2003. Expanding portion sizes in the U.S. marketplace: implications for nutrition counseling. *J Am Diet Assoc* 103(2):231–234.

INDEX

THE MARLOWE DIABETES LIBRARY
Good control is in your hands.

Marlowe Diabetes Library titles are available from online and bricks-and-mortar retailers nationally. For more information about the Marlowe Diabetes Library or any of our books or authors, visit www.marlowepub.com/diabeteslibrary or e-mail us at good.control@perseusbooks.com.

The First Year®—Type 2 Diabetes
An Essential Guide for the Newly Diagnosed, 2nd edition
Gretchen Becker | Foreword by Allison B. Goldfine, MD
$16.95

Prediabetes
What You Need to Know to Keep Diabetes Away
Gretchen Becker | Foreword by Allison B. Goldfine, MD
$14.95

The New Glucose Revolution for Diabetes
The Definitive Guide to Managing Diabetes and Prediabetes Using the Glycemic Index
Dr. Jennie Brand-Miller, Kaye Foster-Powell, Dr. Stephen Colagiuri, Alan Barclay
$16.95

The New Glucose Diabetes Revolution Low GI Guide to Diabetes
The Quick Reference Guide to Managing Diabetes Using the Glycemic Index
Dr. Jennie Brand-Miller and Kaye Foster-Powell with Johanna Burani
$6.95

50 Secrets of the Longest Living People with Diabetes
Sheri R. Colberg, PhD, and Steven V. Edelman, MD
$14.99

The 7 Step Diabetes Fitness Plan
Living Well and Being Fit with Diabetes, No Matter Your Weight
Sheri R. Colberg, PhD | Foreword by Anne Peters, MD
$15.95

Eating for Diabetes
A Handbook and Cookbook—with More than 125 Delicious, Nutritious Recipes to Keep You Feeling Great and Your Blood Glucose in Check
Jane Frank
$15.95

Type 1 Diabetes
A Guide for Children, Adolescents, Young Adults—and Their Caregivers
Ragnar Hanas, MD, PhD | Forewords by Stuart Brink, MD, and Jeff Hitchcock
$24.95

Know Your Numbers, Outlive Your Diabetes
Five Essential Health Factors You Can Master to Enjoy a Long and Healthy Life
Richard A. Jackson, MD, and Amy Tenderich
$14.95

Insulin Pump Therapy Demystified
An Essential Guide for Everyone Pumping Insulin
Gabrielle Kaplan-Mayer | Foreword by Gary Scheiner, MS, CDE
$15.95

Losing Weight with Your Diabetes Medication
How Byetta and Other Drugs Can Help You Lose More Weight than You Ever Thought Possible
David Mendosa | Foreword by Joe Prendergast, MD
$14.99

1,001 Tips for Living Well with Diabetes
Firsthand Advice that Really Works
Judith H. McQuown | Foreword by Harry Gruenspan, MD, PhD
$16.95

Diabetes on Your Own Terms
Janis Roszler, RD, CDE, LD/N
$14.95

Think Like a Pancreas
A Practical Guide to Managing Diabetes with Insulin
Gary Scheiner, MS, CDE | Foreword by Barry Goldstein, MD
$15.95

The Ultimate Guide to Accurate Carb Counting
Gary Scheiner, MS, CDE
$9.95

The Mind-Body Diabetes Revolution
A Proven New Program for Better Blood Sugar Control
Richard S. Surwit, PhD, with Alisa Bauman
$14.95